Mark S. Gold, MD
Editor

Eating Disorders, Overeating, and Pathological Attachment to Food: Independent or Addictive Disorders?

Eating Disorders, Overeating, and Pathological Attachment to Food: Independent or Addictive Disorders? has been co-published simultaneously as *Journal of Addictive Diseases*, Volume 23, Number 3 2004.

Pre-publication
REVIEWS,
COMMENTARIES,
EVALUATIONS . . .

"FEW BOOKS CHANGE THE PARA-DIGM FOR MAJOR HEALTH PROBLEMS. MARK GOLD, MD, HAS EDITED ONE OF THOSE ESPECIALLY VALUABLE BOOKS. Putting the tag 'addiction' on obesity opens up hopeful new avenues of research and treatment as it changes the way the disorder is understood. This book lays out the case for calling eating disorders addictions by relating this form of addiction to those that are more familiar. This perspective not only improves the understanding of eating disorders, but also sheds useful new light on alcohol, other drug, and tobacco addictions."

Robert L. DuPont, MD
President
Institute for Behavior & Health, Inc.
Former Director
National Institute on Drug Abuse
Author
The Selfish Brain: Learning from Addiction

More pre-publication
REVIEWS, COMMENTARIES, EVALUATIONS . . .

"IMPORTANT. . . . Dr. Gold, a brilliant addictions researcher, has put together A FIRST-RATE TEAM OF AUTHORS AND SCIENTISTS to tackle this important problem from a multidisciplinary point of view. The text is well organized and includes current references. The hypotheses generated in the text are challenging and interesting. Kudos to Dr. Gold and his excellent team of authors."

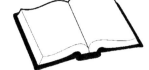

Mark D. Aronson, MD
Professor of Medicine
Harvard Medical School
Vice Chair for Quality
Department of Medicine
Associate Chief
Division of General Medicine
& Primary Care
Beth Israel Deaconess Medical Center
Boston

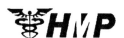

The Haworth Medical Press
An Imprint of The Haworth Press, Inc.

Eating Disorders, Overeating, and Pathological Attachment to Food: Independent or Addictive Disorders?

Eating Disorders, Overeating, and Pathological Attachment to Food: Independent or Addictive Disorders? has been co-published simultaneously as *Journal of Addictive Diseases*, Volume 23, Number 3 2004.

The *Journal of Addictive Diseases* Monographic "Separates"
(formerly *Advances in Alcohol & Substance Abuse* series)*

Below is a list of "separates," which in serials librarianship means a special issue simultaneously published as a special journal issue or double-issue *and* as a "separate" hardbound monograph. (This is a format which we also call a "DocuSerial.")

"Separates" are published because specialized libraries or professionals may wish to purchase a specific thematic issue by itself in a format which can be separately cataloged and shelved, as opposed to purchasing the journal on an on-going basis. Faculty members may also more easily consider a "separate" for classroom adoption.

"Separates" are carefully classified separately with the major book jobbers so that the journal tie-in can be noted on new book order slips to avoid duplicate purchasing.

You may wish to visit Haworth's website at . . .

http://www.HaworthPress.com

. . . to search our online catalog for complete tables of contents of these separates and related publications.

You may also call 1-800-HAWORTH (outside US/Canada: 607-722-5857), or Fax 1-800-895-0582 (outside US/Canada: 607-771-0012), or e-mail at:

docdelivery@haworthpress.com

Eating Disorders, Overeating, and Pathological Attachment to Food: Independent or Addictive Disorders?, edited by Mark S. Gold, MD (Vol. 23, No. 3, 2004). *Examines the relationship between overeating and substance abuse to support the hypothesis that some eating disorders are similar to addiction disorders.*

Addiction Treatment Matching: Research Foundations of the American Society of Addiction Medicine (ASAM) Criteria, edited by David R. Gastfriend, MD (Vol. 22 Suppl. 1, 2003). *Focuses on the ins and outs of the ASAM Criteria–the state-of-the-art in addictions placement matching.*

Effects of Substance Abuse Treatment on AIDS Risk Behaviors, edited by Edward Gottheil, MD, PhD (Vol. 17, No. 4, 1998). *In this important book, you will discover drug abuse treatment methods that will reduce the number of injection episodes and reduce injection use in higher risk settings, such as shooting galleries, thereby reducing your clients risk of infection.*

Smoking and Illicit Drug Use, edited by Mark S. Gold, MD (Vol. 17, No. 1, 1998). *"Based on an understanding of the brain biology of reward, Gold and his colleagues provide policymakers, clinicians, and the public with the best-ever look at the reason why 90% of the nation's more than 60 million cigarette smokers want to quit but have trouble achieving that life-saving goal." (Robert L. DuPont, MD, President, Institute for Behavior and Health, and Professor of Psychiatry, Georgetown University School of Medicine, Rockville, MD). Focuses on the addictive properties of the numerous constituents of tobacco smoke and nicotine dependency.*

The Integration of Pharmacological and Nonpharmacological Treatments in Drug/Alcohol Addictions, edited by Norman S. Miller, MD, and Barry Stimmel, MD (Vol. 16, No. 4, 1997). *Summarizes and provides the groundwork for future considerations in developing and integrating medications with the standard of care for addictions treatment.*

Intensive Outpatient Treatment for the Addictions, edited by Edward Gottheil, MD, PhD (Vol. 16, No. 2, 1997). *"An invaluable source of up-to-date information on important issues relating to IOP, including the active ingredients of successful IOP, the effectiveness of IOP, causes of early dropout, and the impact of psychiatric status and motivation for change on outcomes for patients." (Stephen Magura, PhD, Director, Institute for Treatment Research, National Development & Research institutes, Inc., New York)*

The Neurobiology of Cocaine Addiction: From Bench to Bedside, edited by Herman Joseph, PhD, and Barry Stimmel, MD (Vol. 15, No. 4, 1997). *"Provides an excellent overview of advances in the treatment of cocaine addiction." (The Annals of Pharmacotherapy)*

The Effectiveness of Social Interventions for Homeless Substance Abusers, edited by Gerald J. Stahler, PhD, and Barry Stimmel, MD (Vol. 14, No. 4, 1996). *"Any policymaker or administrator seeking to have a positive impact on the complex problems of this population would be well-advised to thoroughly digest the contents of this volume." (Journal of Behavioral Health Services & Research (formerly the Journal of Mental Health Administration))*

Experimental Therapeutics in Addiction Medicine, edited by Stephen Magura, PhD, and Andrew Rosenblum, PhD (Vol. 13, No. 3/4, 1995). *"Recommended for any clinician involved in caring for patients with substance abuse problems and for those interested in furthering research in this discipline." (The Annals of Pharmacotherapy)*

Comorbidity of Addictive and Psychiatric Disorders, edited by Norman S. Miller, MD (Vol. 12, No. 3, 1993). *"A wealth of factual information . . . it should be included in the library of every psychiatric hospital because it is an excellent reference book." (Israel Journal of Psychiatry)*

Cocaine: Physiological and Physiopathological Effects, edited by Alfonso Paredes, MD, and David A. Gorlick, MD, PhD (Vol. 11, No. 4, 1993). *"The broad range of psychiatric and medical consequences of the epidemic of cocaine use described in this volume should jolt everyone toward increasing strategies to educate, motivate, and stimulate health practitioners at all levels." (Perspectives on Addictions Nursing)*

What Works in Drug Abuse Epidemiology, edited by Blanche Frank, PhD, and Ronald Simeone, PhD (Vol. 11, No. 1, 1992). *"An excellent reference text not only for researchers and scholars, but also for administrators, policymakers, law enforcements agents, and health educators who value the importance of research in decisionmaking at both the micro and macro levels of the ever-growing substance abuse speciality." (International Journal of Epidemiology)*

Cocaine, AIDS, and Intravenous Drug Use, edited by Samuel R. Friedman, PhD, and Douglas S. Lipton, PhD (Vol. 10, No. 4, 1991). *"Examines what has been successful in treatment and prevention and raises issues to promote greater research in the fields for improved treatment and prevention of drug abuse and HIV-infection." (Sci-Tech Book News)*

Behavioral and Biochemical Issues in Substance Abuse, edited by Frank R. George, PhD, and Doris Clouet, PhD* (Vol. 10, No. 1/2, 1991). *"An excellent overview of the power of genetic experimental designs, the results that can be generated as well as the cautions that must be observed in this approach." (Contemporary Psychology)*

Addiction Potential of Abused Drugs and Drug Classes, edited by Carlton K. Erikson, PhD, Martin A. Javors, PhD, and William W. Morgan, PhD* (Vol. 9, No. 1/2, 1990). *"A good reference book for anyone who works in the drug abuse field, particularly those who have responsibilities in the area of community education." (Journal of Psychoactive Drugs)*

Alcohol Research from Bench to Bedside, edited by Enoch Gordis, MD, Boris Tabakoff, PhD, and Markku Linnoila, MD, PhD* (Vol. 7, No. 3/4, 1989). *Scientists and clinicians examine the exciting endeavors in science that have produced medical knowledge applicable to a wide spectrum of treatment and prevention efforts.*

AIDS and Substance Abuse, edited by Larry Siegel, MD* (Vol. 7, No. 2, 1988). *"Contributes in a worthwhile fashion to a number of debates." (British Journal of Addiction)*

Pharmacological Issues in Alcohol and Substance Abuse, edited by Barry Stimmel, MD* (Vol. 7, No. 1, 1988). *"Good reference book for the knowledge of the pharmacology of certain drugs used in treating chemically dependent cases." (Anthony B. Radcliffe, MD, Physician in Charge, Chemical Recovery Program, Kaiser, Pontana, California)*

Children of Alcoholics, edited by Margaret Bean-Bayog, MD, and Barry Stimmel, MD* (Vol. 6, No. 4, 1988). *"This comprehensive volume examines significant research and clinical development in this area." (T.H.E. Journal)*

Cocaine: Pharmacology, Addiction, and Therapy, edited by Mark S. Gold, MD, Marc Galanter, MD, and Barry Stimmel, MD* (Vol. 6, No. 2, 1987). *"Diagnosis and treatment methods are also explored in this highly useful and informative book." (Journal of the American Association of Psychiatric Administrators)*

Alcohol and Substance Abuse in Women and Children, edited by Barry Stimmel, MD* (Vol. 5, No. 3, 1986). *Here is a timely volume that examines the problems of substance abuse in women and children, with a particular emphasis on the role played by the family in the development and perpetuation of the problem.*

Controversies in Alcoholism and Substance Abuse, edited by Barry Stimmel, MD* (Vol. 5, No. 1/2, 1986). *"Thorough, well-informed, and up-to-date." (The British Journal of Psychiatry)*

Alcohol and Substance Abuse in Adolescence, edited by Judith S. Brook, EdD, Dan Lettieri, PhD, David W. Brook, MD, and Barry Stimmel, MD* (Vol. 4, No. 3/4, 1985). *"Contains considerable information that would be useful to mental health clinicians and primary care physicians who deal extensively with adolescents." (The New England Journal of Medicine)*

Alcohol and Drug Abuse in the Affluent, edited by Barry Stimmel, MD* (Vol. 4, No. 2, 1984). *"A valuable contribution to drug abuse literature presenting data on a hitherto under-researched population of drug users." (British Journal of Addiction)*

Cultural and Sociological Aspects of Alcoholism and Substance Abuse, edited by Barry Stimmel, MD* (Vol. 4, No. 1, 1984). *Experts explore the relationship of such factors as ethnicity, family, religion, and gender to chemical abuse and address important implications for treatment.*

Dual Addiction: Pharmacological Issues in the Treatment of Concomitant Alcoholism and Drug Abuse, edited by Mary Jeanne Kreek, MD, and Barry Stimmel, MD* (Vol. 3, No. 4, 1984). *"Provides a good overview of dual addiction." (Contemporary Psychology)*

Conceptual Issues in Alcoholism and Substance Abuse, edited by Joyce H. Lowinson, MD, and Barry Stimmel, MD* (Vol. 3, No. 3, 1984). *This timely volume emphasizes the relevance of current, basic research to the clinical management of the substance abuser.*

The Addictive Behaviors, edited by Howard Shaffer, PhD, and Barry Stimmel, MD* (Vol. 3, No. 1/2, 1984). *"Remarkable . . . is the book's capacity to illustrate social myths and models, to challenge them, and to direct substance abuse professionals in their clinical and research inquiries." (Journal of Psychoactive Drugs)*

Psychosocial Constructs of Alcoholism and Substance Abuse, edited by Barry Stimmel, MD* (Vol. 2, No. 4, 1983). *"An excellent vehicle for orienting interested readers toward critical reference materials and important psychosocial issues." (Bulletin of the Society of Psychologists in Addictive Behaviors)*

Federal Priorities in Funding Alcohol and Drug Abuse Programs, edited by Barry Stimmel, MD* (Vol. 2, No. 3, 1983). *Reveals and evaluates current federal funding for chemical abuse treatment problems.*

Current Controversies in Alcoholism, edited by Barry Stimmel, MD* (Vol. 2, No. 2, 1983). *"Articles vary from reports of sophisticated research to essays backed by thorough literature reviews." (Choice)*

Evaluation of Drug Treatment Programs, edited by Barry Stimmel, MD* (Vol. 2, No. 1, 1983). *"Provides the reader with a unique perspective on the effectiveness of drug treatment programs." (American Journal of Pharmaceutical Education)*

Effects of Maternal Alcohol and Drug Abuse on the Newborn, edited by Barry Stimmel, MD* (Vol. 1, No. 3/4, 1982). *"Authoritative and thought-provoking . . . should be carefully studied by those responsible for the management of drug addiction, and especially by obstetricians and neonatal pediatricians." (The British Journal of Psychiatry)*

Recent Advances in the Biology of Alcoholism, edited by Charles S. Lieber, MD, and Barry Stimmel, MD* (Vol. 1, No. 2, 1982). *"A very valuable handbook for researchers and clinicians interested in alcohol metabolism and its interaction with other drugs, and the endocrine system." (Journal of Studies on Alcohol)*

Opiate Receptors, Neurotransmitters, and Drug Dependence: Basic Science-Clinical Correlates, edited by Barry Stimmel, MD* (Vol. 1, No. 1, 1981). *"An exciting, extensive, and innovative approach to the scientific literature in this area." (Journal of Psychoactive Drugs)*

Eating Disorders, Overeating, and Pathological Attachment to Food: Independent or Addictive Disorders?

Mark S. Gold, MD
Editor

Eating Disorders, Overeating, and Pathological Attachment to Food: Independent or Addictive Disorders? has been co-published simultaneously as *Journal of Addictive Diseases*, Volume 23, Number 3 2004.

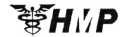

The Haworth Medical Press®
An Imprint of The Haworth Press, Inc.

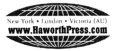

New York • London • Victoria (AU)
www.HaworthPress.com

Published by

The Haworth Medical Press®, 10 Alice Street, Binghamton, NY 13904-1580 USA

The Haworth Medical Press® is an imprint of The Haworth Press, Inc., 10 Alice Street, Binghamton, NY 13904-1580 USA.

Eating Disorders, Overeating, and Pathological Attachment to Food: Independent or Addictive Disorders? has been co-published simultaneously as *Journal of Addictive Diseases*, Volume 23, Number 3 2004.

© 2004 by The Haworth Press, Inc. All rights reserved. No part of this work may be reproduced or utilized in any form or by any means, electronic or mechanical, including photocopying, microfilm and recording, or by any information storage and retrieval system, without permission in writing from the publisher. Printed in the United States of America.

The development, preparation, and publication of this work has been undertaken with great care. However, the publisher, employees, editors, and agents of The Haworth Press and all imprints of The Haworth Press, Inc., including The Haworth Medical Press® and Pharmaceutical Products Press®, are not responsible for any errors contained herein or for consequences that may ensue from use of materials or information contained in this work. Opinions expressed by the author(s) are not necessarily those of The Haworth Press, Inc. With regard to case studies, identities and circumstances of individuals discussed herein have been changed to protect confidentiality. Any resemblance to actual persons, living or dead, is entirely coincidental.

Cover design by Lora Wiggins

Library of Congress Cataloging-in-Publication Data

Eating disorders, overeating, and pathological attachment to food : independent or addictive disorders? / Mark S. Gold, editor.
     p. ; cm.
     "Co-published simultaneously as Journal of addictive diseases, volume 23, number 3 2004."
     Includes bibliographical references and index.
     ISBN 0-7890-2593-0 (hard cover : alk. paper) – ISBN 0-7890-2600-7 (soft cover : alk. paper)
     1. Eating disorders. 2. Compulsive eating. 3. Appetite disorders. 4. Food–Psychological aspects.
     [DNLM: 1. Eating Disorders–etiology. 2. Behavior, Addictive. WM 175 E14815 2004] I. Gold, Mark S.
RC552.E18E2858 2004
616.85'26–dc22
                                         2004006244

Indexing, Abstracting & Website/Internet Coverage

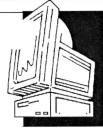

Journal of Addictive Diseases

This section provides you with a list of major indexing & abstracting services. That is to say, each service began covering this periodical during the year noted in the right column. Most Websites which are listed below have indicated that they will either post, disseminate, compile, archive, cite or alert their own Website users with research-based content from this work. (This list is as current as the copyright date of this publication.)

Abstracting, Website/Indexing Coverage . . . . Year When Coverage Began

- *Abstracts in Anthropology* **1991**
- *ADDICTION ABSTRACTS*
  <http://www.tandf.co.uk/addiction-abs> **1994**
- *AgeLine Database <http://research.aarp.org/ageline>* **2000**
- *Behavioral Medicine Abstracts* **1996**
- *Biosciences Information Service of Biological Abstracts
  (BIOSIS) <http://www.biosis.org>* **1983**
- *Business Source Corporate: coverage of nearly 3,350 quality
  magazines and journals; designed to meet the diverse
  information needs of corporations; EBSCO Publishing
  <http://www.epnet.com/corporate/bsourcecorp.asp>* **2003**
- *Cambridge Scientific Abstracts (Health & Safety Science
  Abstracts/Risk Abstracts/Toxicology Abstracts)
  <http://www.csa.com>* **1983**
- *Child Development Abstracts & Bibliography (in print & online)
  <http://www.ukans.edu>* **1982**
- *CINAHL (Cumulative Index to Nursing & Allied Health
  Literature) <http://www.cinahl.com>* **2001**
- *Criminal Justice Abstracts* **1982**
- *Criminal Justice Periodical Index* **1983**
- *Current Contents/Social & Behavioral Sciences
  <http://www.isinet.com>* **1991**

(continued)

(continued)

*Exact start date to come.

*Special Bibliographic Notes related to special journal issues
(separates) and indexing/abstracting:*

- indexing/abstracting services in this list will also cover material in any "separate" that is co-published simultaneously with Haworth's special thematic journal issue or DocuSerial. Indexing/abstracting usually covers material at the article/chapter level.
- monographic co-editions are intended for either non-subscribers or libraries which intend to purchase a second copy for their circulating collections.
- monographic co-editions are reported to all jobbers/wholesalers/approval plans. The source journal is listed as the "series" to assist the prevention of duplicate purchasing in the same manner utilized for books-in-series.
- to facilitate user/access services all indexing/abstracting services are encouraged to utilize the co-indexing entry note indicated at the bottom of the first page of each article/chapter/contribution.
- this is intended to assist a library user of any reference tool (whether print, electronic, online, or CD-ROM) to locate the monographic version if the library has purchased this version but not a subscription to the source journal.
- individual articles/chapters in any Haworth publication are also available through the Haworth Document Delivery Service (HDDS).

∞ ALL HAWORTH MEDICAL PRESS BOOKS
AND JOURNALS ARE PRINTED
ON CERTIFIED ACID-FREE PAPER

Eating Disorders, Overeating, and Pathological Attachment to Food: Independent or Addictive Disorders?

CONTENTS

ABOUT THE EDITOR

Mark S. Gold, MD, is a Distinguished Professor of Psychiatry, Neuroscience, and Community Health & Family Medicine at the University of Florida College of Medicine. He is also a member of the McKnight Brain Institute. Dr. Gold is Chief of the Addiction Medicine Division in the Department of Psychiatry and the department's Vice-Chair for Education.

Dr. Gold is the University of Florida College of Medicine's 2003 Exemplary Teacher and Teacher of the Year. He is a Distinguished Fellow of the American Psychiatric Association (2003). Dr. Gold and his mentors, Drs. Kleber, Redomond, and Aghajanian, won the prestigious Foundations Fund Prize for groundbreaking research in the neurobiology of addiction and withdrawal. Most recently, he won the 2003 research of the year award from the American Academy of Addiction Medicine (ASAM) for his work on the five-year outcome of physician addiction and recovery.

Dr. Gold has written over 900 medical articles, chapters, and abstracts in health professional journals on a wide variety of psychiatric research subjects. He has authored 12 professional books, including practice guidelines, ASAM core competencies, and medical textbooks for primary care professional. He is the author of 15 general audience books. Dr. Gold is a researcher and inventor who worked for nearly 30 years to develop models for understanding the effects of tobacco and other drugs on the brain and behavior.

In 2002, Dr. Gold Chaired an ASAM annual meeting which debated whether food, a exotic and particularly appealing food, might recruit and activate brain systems that are the targets for drugs of abuse. Drugs and food compete for brain reward sites rather than drugs and sex or other primary drives. Dr. Gold has since developed new treatments for addicts. His work at the University of Florida on the brain systems underlying the effects of opiates led to a new norepinephrine hyperactivity hypothesis for opiate withdrawal. His work on cocaine led to the drug being reclassified as dangerous and addicting.

Dr. Gold is the mentor of many of the nation's current leaders in eating disorders and addiction education and research. He is a Distinguished Alumni and an Honors graduate of the University of Florida College of Medicine where he was an AOA and Faculty Research Award winner. Dr. Gold is a current Alumni Board member and is active in numerous national organizations, including the National Scientific Advisory Board for Media Partnership for a Drug Free America, DARE, the American Council for Drug Education, and PRIDE.

Introduction

Obesity is increasingly being recognized as problem of major public health significance. Overeating and obesity are second only to tobacco in annual associated mortality; almost 300,000 deaths per year. Over 10 years ago, we hypothesized that loss of control over eating, which results in obesity, may be another form of addictive behavior and reported on similarities between overeating and classic descriptions of addictions (Are They Addictions or Just Other Types of Problems? ASAM Symposium-1992). Phenomenological and behavioral similarities between substance abuse disorders and food, as a substance of abuse disorder were compelling. At that time, many were critical of including overeating and obesity as an addiction because there were few scientific studies that had directly compared and studied the relationships between these disorders. Researchers only recently have come to a consensus that obesity is a disease, but the debate continues as to whether it is related to depression, personality disorders or addictions. More than a decade after the first ASAM symposium, we were asked again to address this topic (Are Eating Disorders Addictions? ASAM Symposium 2003-2004). Today there is a convincing convergence of evidence from the bench in neuroscience, to PET and fMRI neuroimaging, to data from clinical experience that support the hypothesis that there are important similarities between overeating highly palatable and hedonic foods and the classic addictions.

If drugs of abuse hijack the brain, as has been suggested, where does this occur? Certainly not through existing pathways for sex or water. Food reward, however, is a prime target. Tobacco causes weight loss, as do cocaine, amphetamine, MDMA, and long-term opiate abuse. Drugs

[Haworth co-indexing entry note]: "Introduction." Gold, Mark S. Co-published simultaneously in *Journal of Addictive Diseases* (The Haworth Medical Press, an imprint of The Haworth Press, Inc.) Vol. 23, No. 3, 2004, pp. 1-3; and: *Eating Disorders, Overeating, and Pathological Attachment to Food: Independent or Addictive Disorders?* (ed: Mark S. Gold) The Haworth Medical Press, an imprint of The Haworth Press, Inc., 2004, pp. 1-3. Single or multiple copies of this article are available for a fee from The Haworth Document Delivery Service [1-800-HAWORTH, 9:00 a.m. - 5:00 p.m. (EST). E-mail address: docdelivery@haworthpress.com].

http://www.haworthpress.com/web/JAD
© 2004 by The Haworth Press, Inc. All rights reserved.
Digital Object Identifer: 10.1300/J069v23n03_01

1

of abuse have powerful effects on eating. The 1960s were known as the decade of sex, drugs, and rock and roll. Food seems to be an afterthought and it may be that it is suppressed by drug-taking. We have speculated that if it quacks you can guess that it is a duck. Starving animals self-administer drugs more avidly than those satiated with a good meal or two. Similarly, the wisdom of Alcoholics Anonymous tells us that addicts trying to avoid relapse, should never get too hungry. In this special issue, basic researchers show the relationships between eating messengers and targets for drugs of abuse and the possible inter-connections. Imaging studies show that the brain's somatosensory cortex changes with overeating and obesity so that the mouth and tongue increase their geographical area on the homunculus. Also, the hypothalamus senses that eating has occurred with a delay time that increases with increased body mass. Both these findings, by Dr. Wang and also Dr. Lui reported here, show how increased weight makes further increases more likely. In weight management and bariatric surgery clinics, it is commonly observed that the heavier the patient the less alcohol and illegal drugs they use. It is almost as if they are competing for the same reward sites in the brain. If this is the case, we might see an effect of drug treatment on weight. Treatment of addicts appears to result in weight gain. Not just smoking cessation but all supervised drug abstinence treatment causes weight gain. Here numerous researchers examine the links between overeating, obesity, and addictions in an attempt to answer the question: Are Eating Disorders Addictions?

Kalra and Kalra show the relationships between eating messengers and targets for drugs of abuse and the possible inter-connections in their paper entitled, "Overlapping and Interactive Pathways Regulating Appetite and Craving." Other imaging studies, such as the fMRI study by Dr. Liu and colleagues entitled, "Interaction of Satiety and Reward Response to Food Stimulation," show that the hypothalamus senses that eating has occurred with a delay time that increases with increased body mass. Imaging studies, such as reported by Dr. Wang and colleagues show that the brain's somatosensory cortex changes with overeating and obesity so that the mouth and tongue increase their geographical area on the homunculus. Wang and colleagues report on "Similarity Between Obesity and Drug Addiction as Assessed by Neurofunctional Imaging: A Concept Review," in this issue.

In "Adolescent Drug Addiction Treatment and Weight Gain," Dr. Hodgkins et al. report that weight gain follows supervised abstinence from drugs and alcohol. In the next article, "Examining Problem Drinking and Eating Disorders from a Gendered Perspective," Matthews examines problem drinking and eating disorders in a college student population. Males were more likely to report problem drinking whereas women were more likely to report symptoms of eating disorders. In their study, only a small subset of female subjects had both problem drinking and eating disorder symptomatology. As they predicted, they did find a significant relationship between problem drinking and higher scores on the Impulse Regulation subscale of the Eating Disorder Inventory-2.

In the next article, Anne Becker and colleagues review the social and genetic factors related to eating disorders in "Genes and/or Jeans?: Genetic and Socio-Cultural Contributions to Risk for Eating Disorders." It appears there are numerous complex genetic and environmental etiologic mechanisms. Genetic studies have focused on anorexia nervosa more often than binge-eating or bulimia nervosa, but recent studies are demonstrating that they may be etiologically separate. In the final paper, we report that as BMI increases, alcohol use decreases. It is possible they compete for reward sites in the brain and therefore we would expect to see weight gain after substance abuse treatment.

Over a decade ago, we reported on the similarities of overeating and obesity to classic addictions. Since that time, neuroimaging studies have supported the hypothesis that loss of control over eating and obesity produces changes in the brain, which are similar to those produced by drugs of abuse. In addition, newly discovered messengers such as leptin, galanin, CART have effects in modulating eating behavior and may have roles in alcohol and other drug dependencies. Treatment of obesity, from surgery to medications, often involves 12-step meetings. Overeating and obesity are increasing in prevalence and public health significance. Applying research methodologies applied to addictions may offer hope for understanding and the development of common treatments.

Some would say if it quacks like a duck, it is a duck. Food, highly palatable and energy dense, has become a substance of abuse. Overeating and obesity may be readily included in the DSM-IV by simply considering food as a "substance" in SUDs. Loss of control, use despite diabetes and other consequences, changing priorities and so on would make criteria for SUD.

Mark S. Gold, MD
Departments of Psychiatry and Neuroscience
McKnight Brain Institute
University of Florida
Gainesville, FL 32610

Overlapping and Interactive Pathways Regulating Appetite and Craving

Satya P. Kalra, PhD
Pushpa S. Kalra, PhD

SUMMARY. Multidisciplinary research in recent years has delineated the hypothalamic hardcore wiring that encodes appetitive drive. The appetite regulating network (ARN) consisting of distinct orexigenic and anorexigenic circuitries operates in the arcuate nucleus–paraventricular nucleus axis of the hypothalamus to propagate and relay the appetitive drive, and is subject to modulation by excitatory and inhibitory messages from the lateral hypothalamus and ventromedial nucleus, respectively. Reciprocal afferent humoral signals, comprised of anorexigenic leptin from white adipose tissue and orexigenic ghrelin from stomach, to the ARN integrate the moment-to-moment regulation of energy homeostasis. Various loci in the ARN and afferent hormonal feedback circuitry in the rodent brain are important for food craving elicited by drugs of abuse. This convergence of neurochemical and hormonal signaling has

Satya P. Kalra, Department of Neuroscience, University of Florida McKnight Brain Institute, Gainesville, FL, USA (E-mail: skalra@ufbi.ufl.edu).

Pushpa S. Kalra, Department of Physiology & Functional Genomics, University of Florida McKnight Brain Institute, Gainesville, FL, USA

Address correspondence to: Satya P. Kalra, PhD, University of Florida McKnight Brain Institute, Department of Neuroscience, P.O. Box 100244, Gainesville, FL 32610-0244.

This research was supported by the National Institute of Health (DK37273 and NS32727). The authors wish to acknowledge Ms. Sandra Clark for word processing assistance.

[Haworth co-indexing entry note]: "Overlapping and Interactive Pathways Regulating Appetite and Craving." Kalra, Satya P., and Pushpa S. Kalra. Co-published simultaneously in *Journal of Addictive Diseases* (The Haworth Medical Press, an imprint of The Haworth Press, Inc.) Vol. 23, No. 3, 2004, pp. 5-21; and: *Eating Disorders, Overeating, and Pathological Attachment to Food: Independent or Addictive Disorders?* (ed: Mark S. Gold) The Haworth Medical Press, an imprint of The Haworth Press, Inc., 2004, pp. 5-21. Single or multiple copies of this article are available for a fee from The Haworth Document Delivery Service [1-800-HAWORTH, 9:00 a.m. - 5:00 p.m. (EST). E-mail address: docdelivery@haworthpress.com].

http://www.haworthpress.com/web/JAD
© 2004 by The Haworth Press, Inc. All rights reserved.
Digital Object Identifer: 10.1300/J069v23n03_02

now paved the way to address the fundamental question of whether cellular and molecular events that underlie the appetitive drive in response to diminished energy stores in the body are akin to drug craving during withdrawl in humans. *[Article copies available for a fee from The Haworth Document Delivery Service: 1-800-HAWORTH. E-mail address: <docdelivery@ haworthpress.com> Website: <http://www.HaworthPress.com> © 2004 by The Haworth Press, Inc. All rights reserved.]*

KEYWORDS. Appetite, circuitry, hypothalamus, neuropeptide Y, opiates, leptin, ghrelin, hormones, addiction, craving, nicotine, ethanol, endocannabinoids

INTRODUCTION

The hypothalamus has been recognized for over a century as the primary site in the central nervous system (CNS) for integration of internal and external environmental information for energy homeostasis.[1,2] Research conducted between 1940-1980 suggested daily regulation of weight homeostasis by a "dual" center, ventromedial medial hypothalamus (VMH) as the "satiety" and lateral hypothalamus (LH) as the "hunger" center.[1-3] This neuroanatomical landscape changed dramatically after the discovery in 1984 of a 36 amino acid peptide, Neuropeptide Y (NPY), as the most potent appetite transducer. Produced in the arcuate nucleus (ARC), its target sites are located in the paraventricular nucleus (PVN) and neighboring sites in the hypothalamus.[1,4,5] This new insight not only shifted the focus of research from the classic unifying dual center anatomical base to the ARC-PVN as the primary neuroaxis that propagates and relays the appetitive drive, but also sparked intense research that unraveled an interactive appetite regulating network (ARN) spanning multiple hypothalamic sites and a diverse array of neurotransmitters/neuromodulators.[2] Isolation of the adipocyte hormone leptin as an anorexigenic peripheral hormonal signal a decade later, and recently of ghrelin produced by oxyntic cells of the stomach, as an orexigenic hormonal signal,[6-9] provided the key players in the feedback circuitry between ARN and peripheral visceral organs for energy homeostasis.[2,10] Research in the past three decades also focused on identifying the neurochemical pathways that encode craving and addiction for drugs of abuse.[11,12] The discovery in the 1970s of opiate receptors, binding sites for endogenous opioid peptides (EOP) in mediating opiate addiction, strengthened the notion that distinct neurochemical modalities that encode craving exist in the CNS.[11-13] However, reports that all three classes of EOP–β-endorphin, enkephalins, and dynorphin–are produced in hypothalamic sites implicated in regulation of appetite and, like the opiate morphine,[2,13] each of these EOP stimulated feeding,[14] hinted early on at the existence of cross talk between the networks regulating appetite and craving for reward and pleasure. Suppression of NPY-induced feeding by opiate receptor antagonists[14] and the existence of morphological links between NPY and β-endorphin producing neurons,[2,15] corroborated this implied functional association. The list of drugs of abuse that are likely to affect energy intake by modulating the ARN has grown in the last decade.[16]

In this article, first we have reviewed briefly the current knowledge of the ARN and the feedback regulatory loop between peripheral hormonal signals and ARN, and then collated experimental evidence to illustrate the role of key players in the ARN in linking craving for food elicited by drugs of abuse.

HYPOTHALAMIC REGULATION OF APPETITE

Neuroanatomical Substrate

Five discrete sites in the hypothalamus have been shown to participate in regulation of food intake and energy expenditure.[2] The orexigenic and anorexigenic signal molecues are synthesized in discrete subpopulations of neurons in the ARC and released at target sites in the two subdivisions of the PVN, the parvocellular PVN (pPVN) and magnocellular PVN (mPVN, Figure 1). Synthesis and release of these neurotransmitters in the ARC-PVN axis is, in turn, modulated by the ventromedial nucleus (VMN) and lateral hypothalamus (LH). Disruption in communication between these two sites resulted in unabated hyperphagia and abnormal weight gain suggesting that the VMN relays inhibitory information to the ARC.[2] However, the neurotransmitter(s) involved is unknown. On the other hand, discrete subpopulations of neurons in the LH, expressing orexin (ORX) or melanin concentrating hormone (MCH), stimulate appetite by increasing NPY signaling in the ARC-PVN axis.[2,17-19] In addition, recent studies have shown that sympathetic nervous system fibres emanating from the medial preoptic area (MPOA) and traversing caudally through the PVN enroute to the brown

FIGURE 1. A diagrammatic representation of hypothalamic circuitry regulating appetite under the regulatory feedback control of afferent hormonal signals, anorexigenic leptin from white adipose tissue and orexigenic ghrelin from stomach. The orexigenic pathway consists of NPY, GABA and AgrP co-expressing neurons in the arcuate nucleus (ARC) of the hypothalamus. These neurochemical signals stimulate appetite by an action at target sites in the paraventricular nucleus (PVN), and by restraining the appetite inhibiting effects of melanocortin pathway consisting of POMC and CART coexpressing neurons in the ARC. In addition, MCH and ORX expressing neurons located in the lateral hypothalamus (LH) stimulate appetite by enhancing NPYergic signaling in the ARC-PVN axis. The unidentified neuronal populations in the ventromedial nucleus exert an inhibitory influence on the appetite regulating circuitry in the ARC-PVN axis. Leptin exerts a tonic restraint on appetite by inhibiting orexigenic NPY signaling and enhancing melanocortin signaling in the ARC-PVN axis. Ghrelin stimulates appetite by increasing orexigenic NPYergic signaling in the ARC-PVN axis. Numbers in circles depict the loci of action of drugs of abuse in the appetite regulating hypothalamic circuitry. (+) = excitatory, (−) = inhibitory, (?) = unknown neuronal phenotype. For details see text.

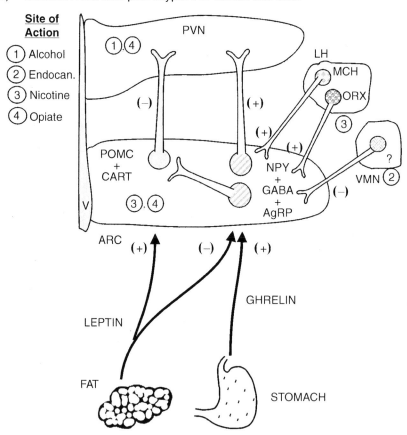

adipose tissue (BAT) in the periphery regulate thermogenic energy expenditure, an essential component in energy homeostasis.[20]

APPETITE REGULATING NETWORKS

Orexigenic Pathways

It is well established that the primary orexigenic pathway in the hypothalamus originates from a subpopulation of neurons in the ARC that coexpress NPY, agouti related peptide (AgrP) and γ-aminobutyric acid (GABA). When released in the PVN, these three neurotransmitters act in disparate ways. NPY stimulates food intake by activation of NPY Y1 and Y5 receptors in the mPVN[2] (Figure 1). Continuous stimulation of NPY receptors produced relentless hyperphagia, increased the rate of body weight gain and culminated in morbid obesity.[2,21] Interestingly, there was no evidence of development of either tolerance or receptor down-regulation despite sustained NPY receptor activation.[21] Both fasting and dieting readily increased NPY synthesis in the ARC and release in the PVN to sustain the appetitive drive needed for energy replenishment.[2,22] Interestingly, diminution in NPY availability at target sites in the PVN and possibly in the ARC enhanced NPY Y1 receptor sensitivity to the extent that these rats also displayed hyperphagia and overt obesity.[2,23] Seemingly, imbalance in NPY signaling locally in the ARC and PVN results in unregulated phagia involving distinctive molecular sequalae.

GABA has been shown to stimulate feeding via GABA^A receptor activation, a response that can be enhanced when it is coadministered with NPY.[24] It seems that it is the dampening of the tonic restraint by GABA in the pPVN augments stimulation of appetite by NPY. In addition, there is evidence to show that GABA release locally in the ARC itself may reduce anorexigenic melanocortin signaling to the PVN, resulting in enhanced feeding.[25] In contrast to GABA, the third co-expressed orexigenic peptide AgrP, stimulates feeding by yet another mode of signal relay in the PVN. AgrP is an endogenous antagonist at melanocortin 4 (MC4) receptors, the receptor that mediates the tonic restrain on feeding.[2,26,27] Taken together, it seems that a two prong action, direct stimulation of feeding by NPY along with the GABA and AgrP-induced curb on the restraint on feeding propagates the appetitive drive. Recent morphological evidence of co-expression of NPY Y1 and Y5, GABA^A and

MC4 receptors and electrophysiological demonstrations of the interplay among these varied messengers in the PVN corroborated the suggestion that the ARC-PVN axis is the final common orexigenic pathway involved in regulation of NPY-induced appetite[2,10,28,29] (Figure 1).

Fiber projections from the LH, in contrast to those from the VMN, relay excitatory information to the ARC-PVN axis[2] (Figure 1). Central administration of ORX or MCH stimulated feeding but to a far lesser extent than that evoked by NPY, and interestingly, prior administration of Y1 and Y5 receptor antagonists blocked the ORX- and MCH-induced feeding.[30-32] Thus, the excitatory effects of these two neuropeptides produced in the LH are apparently mediated by NPY pathway. Morphological evidence of synaptic links between the ORX- and MCH-expressing neurons in the LH with NPY neurons in the ARC supports this mode of LH involvement.[33,34] In addition, since fasting increased gene expression and release of NPY in the ARC-PVN axis, and augmented gene expression of ORX and MCH in the LH, it is highly likely that these LH afferents to the ARC augment NPY signaling in the ARC-PVN axis. Overall, LH neurons expressing ORX and MCH and ARC neurons coexpressing NPY, AgrP and GABA apparently constitute the hard core wiring of the orexigenic network in the hypothalamus. Further, it is also likely that ascending afferent messages from visceral organs and from the mesolimbic reward pathway are relayed to the ARC-PVN axis by these peptidergic pathways emanating from the LH.

Anorexigenic Pathways

Two distinct hypothalamic anorexigenic neural pathways are the likely candidates in transmitting an inhibitory control on appetite. The physiologically relevant one is the melanocortin pathway in the ARC-PVN axis.[2,25,28] As mentioned in the foregoing section, POMC neurons in the ARC coexpress the anorexigenic peptides, α-MSH and cocaine- and amphetamine-regulating transcript (CART, Figure 1). Various lines of evidence suggested that these peptides are released in the PVN where they act to inhibit feeding.[2,25,28] The inhibitory effects of α-MSH are mediated by MC4 receptors. That these receptors normally mediate the tonic restraint on feeding is evidenced by the development hyperphagia and obesity in mice with a null mutation for MC4 receptors.[2,25,35] Fasting decreased POMC gene expression and α-MSH release.[2,35,36] Since CART also inhibited feeding, one can assume that a concerted action of CART and α-MSH is a physiologically relevant anorexigenic signal.[2,25,35,36] The other anorexigenic pathway, consisting of corticotropin releasing hormone (CRH) expressing neurons, has been studied extensively for its involvement in stress-related impacts on appetite.[14,36] In contrast to POMC neurons, these neurons are located in the PVN and presumably, CRH released locally in PVN mediates the stress-induced inhibition of food intake. Although CRH can inhibit NPY-induced food intake, the ARC NPY neurons have been shown to stimulate CRH release,[2,14] an observation not in keeping with a physiological role of CRH in regulation of appetite on a daily basis.

Overall, existence of synaptic links between NPY and POMC neurons in the ARC, and between NPY and CRH neurons in the PVN, electrophysiological findings affirming communication between NPY and POMC neurons in the ARC, and evidence that α-MSH, CART, and CRH can inhibit NPY-induced feeding, reveal the intricate interplay among various players in the hypothalamic anorexigenic and orexigenic circuitries in the daily patterning of ingestive behavior (Figure 1).

REGULATION OF THE HYPOTHALAMIC APPETITE REGULATING NETWORK BY AFFERENT HORMONAL SIGNALS

It is now apparent that the peripheral hormones–leptin from adipocytes, and ghrelin from stomach–modulate the moment-to-moment operation of the hypothalamic ARN (Figure 1). Leptin and ghrelin can cross the blood brain barrier to gain access to targets sites in the hypothalamus.[2,6,8] In addition, leptin and ghrelin are also expressed in distinct subpopulations of neurons in the hypothalamus.[37,38] There is general consensus that leptin exerts a tonic restraint on feeding by activating the biologically active long-form of leptin receptors expressed in NPY, ORX, and β-endorphin plus α-MSH producing POMC neurons in the hypothalamus.[2,6,36] A decrease in blood leptin levels, either during the pre-meal interval or in response to fasting and food restriction, sets in motion a chain of neural events in the hypothalamic ARN that elicit orexigenic NPY, AgrP, and GABA secretion in concert with diminution in anorexigenic α-MSH release in the PVN. This simultaneous two prong action, increased orexigenic and decreased anorexigenic signaling in the ARC-PVN axis facilitates the appetitive drive.[2,10,20]

Recently, ghrelin has also been shown to play a prominent role in stimulation of appetite.[7-10] Blood ghrelin levels increase in the pre-meal interval and in response to fasting. Ghrelin administration stimulated feeding and repeated daily injections promoted adiposity. Stimulation of feeding by ghrelin is mediated by the NPY pathway in the ARC-PVN axis.[8,9] Our investigations revealed a dynamic interplay between leptin and ghrelin, in which leptin plays a dual regulatory control on appetite expression.[10,20] We observed that leptin suppressed ghrelin secretion from the stomach and antagonized the excitatory effects of ghrelin on feeding by an action at the level of ARC NPY neurons in the hypothalamus.[20,39-42] Based on these recent findings together with the mounting evidence of a crucial central action of each of these afferent hormonal signals, we proposed that a reciprocal interplay of inhibitory leptin and excitatory ghrelin feedback on the ARN is responsible for sustaining energy homeostasis on a daily basis.[10,20]

On the other hand, extensive evidence from clinical and basic research showed that increased energy storage in the body resulting from consumption of a diet rich in calories and/or decreased energy expenditure due to a sedentary life style, promoted hyperleptinemia in proportion to increased fat accretion.[2,6,43,44] Seemingly, due to restricted transport of leptin across the blood brain barrier and suboptimal leptin production locally in the hypothalamus, this diet-induced hyperleptinemia is ineffective in curbing food intake and enhance energy expenditure to impose weight homeostasis. A series of investigations from our laboratory has shown that it is possible to circumvent this central leptin insufficiency and restore the leptin restraint within the hypothalamus with the aid of central leptin gene therapy.[39-41,45,46] A single injection into the hypothalamus of recombinant adeno-associated virus vector encoding leptin suppressed age-related weight gain in prepubertal and adult rats and blocked diet-induced obesity. This suppression of weight gain for long periods was associated with depletion of fat depots as a result of a spectrum of neural events that included decreases in orexigenic NPY and increases in anorexigenic melanocortin signaling in the hypothalamus, and increased thermogenic energy expenditure. Seemingly, central gene therapy is a novel therapeutic modality to selectively restore the leptin deficiency within the hypothalamus.[46,47]

CRAVING AND HYPOTHALAMIC APPETITE REGULATING PATHWAYS

Drug addiction is a chronic relapsing brain disorder, an outcome of a host of interacting factors that enhance motivation or craving for substances to achieve an enhanced state of energy, arousal or euphoria. The mesolimbic reward system extending from the ventral tegmentum to the nucleus accumbens with projections to limbic systems and orbital frontal cortex, is apparently one common neural pathway that all licit and illicit drugs employ for positive reinforcement of craving.[11,12,48] A high degree of concurrence of substance abuse and eating disorders–hyperphagia, anorexia, and bulimia–has been reported in humans.[49] The new knowledge of the hypothalamic hardcore wiring for appetitive drive, as briefly described in the preceding sections, has raised the intriguing possibility of a commonality of neurochemical signaling in motivation for food and drug seeking behaviors. In this context, three questions arise: Do the components of the hardcore wiring of the ARN cross talk with that of craving? Are the underpinnings of drug craving during withdrawal similar to the motivational drive for food when faced with insufficient or depleted energy stores? Do addictive drugs mobilize neurochemical modalities in the ARN to elicit anorexia or hyperphagia? What follows is a brief review of the impact of well-known drugs of abuse on the dynamic operation of the ARN in conjunction with modified appetitive behavior, in an attempt to discern the overlapping and interactive mechanisms underlying appetite and craving.

Ethanol

Multidisciplinary approaches have implicated the brain NPY system in alcohol abuse (Figure 1). NPY-deficient mice consume excessive amounts of ethanol and conversely, mice overexpressing NPY in the brain, but not in the hypothalamic ARC, drink less alcohol as compared with wild-type mice.[50-55] Despite the fact that selectively bred alcohol preferring rats display lower levels of NPY in several brain sites, NPY levels in the hypothalamic ARC-PVN axis were augmented as compared to non-preferring rats.[51-53] Similarly, Clark et al.[54] found that consumption of a 6% ethanol diet raised NPY levels in the PVN and modified the feeding pattern. Interestingly, infusion of NPY directly into the PVN increased ethanol self-administration and preference.[55] In contrast, intraventricular NPY injection acutely attenuated the behavioral effects of ethanol withdrawal.[56] Other reports implied involvement of Y1 receptor in regulation of voluntary ethanol consumption.[57] Further, genetic linkage analysis in rats and study of polymorphism in NPY gene in humans suggested a role for NPY in ethanol consumption and in seizure during withdrawal.[52,58] Ethanol consumption has been reported to modify secretion of leptin, the other important component of appetite regulating feedback circuitry and circulating leptin levels have been correlated with chronic ethanol consumption concomitant with no discernible shift in ingestive behavior in mice.[59-61] In summary, whereas various lines of evidence implicate NPY and leptin signalings in alcohol addiction, there is a paucity of definitive information to correlate NPY synthesis and release in the ARC-PVN axis and ethanol consumption and craving, in a manner as delineated for appetite.[2]

Endocannabinoids

A comparative analysis of the effects of various drugs of abuse indicates that endocannabinoids may play a role in the hypothalamic regulation of appetite. Delta-9-tetrahydrocannabinol (Δ^9-THC), an active component of cannabis, stimulates appetite by activating CB1 cannabinoid receptors, and it has found clinical application to improve appetite in patients suffering from cancer or HIV-included cachexia and wasting.[62] Several investigators showed that the endocannabinoids, anadamide and 2-arachidonoyl glycerol, stimulated phagia and levels of endocannabinoids in the hypothalamus increased in obese, hyperphagic rodents deficient in leptin.[63-67] Leptin replacement reduced endocannabinoids along with a reduction in feeding.[65,66] Furthermore, CB1 receptor antagonist decreased food intake in wild type but not in CB1 knock-out mice. Fasting increased and refeeding decreased endogenous cannabinoid levels in the hypothalamus in a fashion similar to the reported shifts in hypothalamic NPY. Microinjection of anadamide into the ventral medial hypothalamus stimulated feeding, although to a lesser extent than that seen after injection in nucleus accumbens shell, a response blocked by CB1 receptor antagonist[68] (Figure 1). Taken together, these findings are suggestive of a role for hypothalamic endocannabinoids in influencing food-intake behavior not only in response to drug challenges but as putative mediators of the tonic restraint on feeding exerted by leptin in a fashion quite similar to that observed for orexigenic NPY, ORX, and MCH.

Nicotine

Because numerous epidemiological studies document a relationship between tobacco smoking and reduced body weight, and weight gain after cessation of smoking,[69,70] there has been an increased interest recently in characterizing the neural and molecular sequalae underlying this inverse relationship between nicotine consumption and weight gain. In rodents, nicotine administration decreased body weight, possibly due to diminished food intake and increased energy expenditure.[71-73] The weight loss is attributable partly to reduced fat deposition because circulating leptin levels decreased concomitantly.[74] However, contrary to expectations, NPY and ORX gene expression in the hypothalamus were enhanced by nicotine, an observation that implied increased availability of orexigenic peptide concomitant with reduced food intake.[71,75,76] Further analysis showed that nicotine injections inhibited NPY Y1 receptors gene expression, a response previously shown to be responsible for inhibition of appetite by leptin and cytokines[77,78] (Figure 1). Furthermore, nicotine, like leptin,[39-41,45] increased UCP1 mRNA in brown adipose tissue, implying increased thermogenic energy expenditure.[72] Therefore, it is highly likely that nicotine-induced weight loss results from reduced appetite imposed by diminution in NPY receptor mediated orexigenic signaling together with increased energy expenditure. Conversely, cessation of smoking apparently reverses these hypothalamic-driven sequalae of events leading to rapid weight regain. On the basis of these findings, we propose that like leptin,[46,78] nicotine restrains weight gain by simultaneously decreasing NPY signaling through NPY Y1 receptors and increasing thermogenic energy expenditure. It is true that, unlike leptin,[22] nicotine increased levels of NPY and ORX in the ARC-PVN axis,[71,76] presumably resulting from diminished circulating leptin levels due to a loss in fat tissue, it concurrently suppressed NPY Y1 receptor abundance, thereby blocking the effectiveness of orexigenic NPY and ORX.[2,76-78]

Opiates

It is well known that opiates, including morphine, promote phagia and EOP stimulate feeding in a receptor and site-specific manner.[14,79] Microinjection of EOP in selected hypothalamic sites stimulated a short-lived, modest increase in feeding that was blocked by selective receptor antagonists.[2,79,80] Since morphological evidence suggested a close association between NPY and β-endorphin and α-MSH expressing POMC neurons in the ARC,[2,15] and NPY stimulated–β-endorphin release and inhibited α-MSH release from the hypothalamus,[2,81] and opiate receptor antagonist suppress NPY and AgrP-induced feeding, it is highly likely that the appetite stimulating effects of opiates and EOP are mediated by the hypothalamic NPY network[79,80,82,83] (Figure 1). Future research towards elucidating intracellular mechanisms that permit differential release of β-endorphin and α-MSH from the ARC POMC neurons should shed light on the physiological relevance of EOP in the hypothalamic integration of feeding behavior on a daily basis and how EOP signaling within the ARN mediates opiate addiction.

CONCLUDING REMARKS

Although the neurobiological processes by which drug craving develops are not fully understood, much progress has been made in recent years towards delineating the anatomical and functional associations between ingestive and drug seeking behaviors. This has been made possible by recent unraveling of the hypothalamic circuitry and internal afferent hormonal signals that drive this neuropeptidergic circuitry for timely expression of appetite on a daily basis. A most revealing outcome is that addictive drugs employ one or more components of the hypothalamic hard core wiring, and/or afferent signaling to affect appetite. Although this finding may account for drug-induced hyperphagia or anorexia, it sheds little light on the question of whether the appetitive drive in response to insufficient energy stores in the body is akin to drug craving during withdrawal. Nevertheless, these findings in rodents are a step forward for concerted research towards a better understanding of the neural basis of craving in humans, which may catalyze the development of new therapeutic options to curb the epidemic of eating disorders and drug addiction.

REFERENCES

1. Bray GA. Historical framework for the development of ideas about obesity. In: Handbook of Obesity, Marcel DeKer, Inc., ed., New York: 1998:1-29.

2. Kalra SP, Dube MG, Pu S, et al. Interacting appetite-regulating pathways in the hypothalamic regulation of body weight. Endocr Rev. 1999;20:68-100.

3. Anand BK, Brobeck JR. Hypothalamic control of food intake in rats and cats. The Yale Journal of Biology and Medicine. 1951;24:123-146.

4. Clark JT, Kalra PS, Crowley WR, Kalra SP. Neuropeptide Y and human pancreatic polypeptide stimulate feeding behavior in rats. Endocrinology. 1984;115:427-429.

5. Kalra SP, Clark JT, Sahu A, et al. Control of feeding and sexual behaviors by neuropeptide Y: Physiological implications. Synapse. 1988;2:254-257.

6. Friedman JM, Halaas JL. Leptin and the regulation of body weight in mammals. Nature. 1998;395:763-770.

7. Kojima M, Hosoda H, Date Y, et al. Ghrelin is a growth-hormone-releasing acylated peptide from stomach. Nature. 1999; 402:656-660.

8. Tschop M, Smiley DL, Heiman ML. Ghrelin induces adiposity in rodents. Nature. 2000;407:908-913.

9. Nakazato M, Murakami N, Date Y, et al. A role for ghrelin in the central regulation of feeding. Nature. 2001;409:194-198.

10. Kalra SP, Bagnasco M, Otukonyong EE, et al. Rhythmic, reciprocal ghrelin and leptin signaling: New insight in the development of obesity. Regul Pept. 2003;111: 1-11.

11. Tartar RE, Ammerman RT, Ott PJ. Handbook of substance abuse. In: Neurobehavioral Pharmacology. Tartar RE, Ammerman RT, Ott PJ eds. New York: Premum Press, 1998.

12. Kalivas PW, Samson HH. The Neurobiology of drug and alcohol addiction. Ann N Y Acad Sci. 1992;654:1-545.

13. Imura H, Kato Y, Nakai Y, et al. Endogenous opioids and related peptides: From molecular biology to clinical medicine. The Sir Henry Dale lecture for 1985. J Endocrinol. 1985;107:147-157.

14. Morley JE. Neuropeptide regulation of appetite and weight. Endocr Rev. 1987; 8:256-287.

15. Horvath TL, Naftolin F, Kalra SP, Leranth C. Neuropeptide-Y innervation of beta-endorphin-containing cells in the rat mediobasal hypothalamus: A light and electron microscopic double immunostaining analysis. Endocrinology. 1992;131:2461-2467.

16. Karch SB. Pathology of Drug Abuse. CRC Press LLC, Boca Raton, FL 2002, pp. 1-537.

17. De Lecea L, Kilduff TS, Peyron C, et al. The hypocretins: Hypothalamus-specific peptides with neuroexcitatory activity. Proc Natl Acad Sci. 1998;95:322-327.

18. Dube MG, Kalra SP, Kalra PS. Food intake elicited by central administration of orexins/hypocretins: Identification of hypothalamic sites of action. Brain Res. 1999; 842:473-477.

19. Qu D, Ludwig DS, Gammeltoft S, et al. A role for melanin-concentrating hormone in the central regulation of feeding behaviour. Nature. 1996;380:243-247.

20. Bagnasco M, Dube MG, Kalra PS, Kalra SP. Evidence for the existence of distinct central appetite and energy expenditure pathways and stimulation of ghrelin as revealed by hypothalamic site-specific leptin gene therapy. Endocrinology. 2002;143: 4409-4421.

21. Kalra SP, Kalra PS. Nutritional infertility: The role of the interconnected hypothalamic neuropeptide Y-galanin-opioid network. Front Neuroendocrinol. 1996;17: 371-401.

22. Kalra SP, Dube MG, Sahu A, et al. Neuropeptide Y secretion increases in the paraventricular nucleus in association with increased appetite for food. Proc Natl Acad Sci. 1991;88:10931-10935.

23. Kalra PS, Dube MG, Xu B, Kalra SP. Increased receptor sensitivity to neuropeptide Y in the hypothalamus may underlie transient hyperphagia and body weight gain. Regul Pept. 1997;72:121-130.

24. Pu S, Jain MR, Horvath TL, et al. Interactions between neuropeptide Y and gamma-aminobutyric acid in stimulation of feeding: A morphological and pharmacological analysis. Endocrinology. 1999;140:933-940.

25. Cowley MA, Smart JL, Rubinstein M, et al. Leptin activates anorexigenic POMC neurons through a neural network in the arcuate nucleus. Nature. 2001; 411:480-484.

26. Ollmann MM, Wilson BD, Yang YK, et al. Antagonism of central melanocortin receptors in vitro and in vivo by agouti-related protein. Science. 1997;278:135-138.

27. Hahn TM, Breininger JF, Baskin DG, Schwartz MW. Coexpression of Agrp and NPY in fasting-activated hypothalamic neurons. Nat Neurosci. 1998;1:271-272.

28. Broberger C, Hokfelt T. Hypothalamic and vagal neuropeptide circuitries regulating food intake. Physiol Behav. 2001;74:669-682.

29. Smith MS, Grove KL. Integration of the regulation of reproductive function and energy balance: Lactation as a model. Front Neuroendocrinol. 2002;23:225-256.

30. Jain MR, Horvath TL, Kalra PS, Kalra SP. Evidence that NPY Y1 receptors are involved in stimulation of feeding by orexins (hypocretins) in sated rats. Regul Pept. 2000;87:19-24.

31. Dube MG, Horvath TL, Kalra PS, Kalra SP. Evidence of NPY Y5 receptor involvement in food intake elicited by orexin A in sated rats. Peptides. 2000;21: 1557-1560.

32. Chaffer CL, Morris MJ. The feeding response to melanin-concentrating hormone is attenuated by antagonism of the NPY Y(1)-receptor in the rat. Endocrinology. 2002;143:191-197.

33. Horvath TL, Diano S, van den Pol AN. Synaptic interaction between hypocretin (orexin) and neuropeptide Y cells in the rodent and primate hypothalamus: A novel circuit implicated in metabolic and endocrine regulations. J Neurosci. 1999;19:1072-1087.

34. Elias CF, Saper CB, Maratos-Flier E, et al. Chemically defined projections linking the mediobasal hypothalamus and the lateral hypothalamic area. J Comp Neurol. 1998;402:442-459.

35. Saper CB, Chou TC, Elmquist JK. The need to feed: Homeostatic and hedonic control of eating. Neuron. 2002;36:199-211.

36. Schwartz MW, Woods SC, Porte D, et al. Central nervous system control of food intake. Nature. 2000;404:661-671.

37. Horvath TL, Diano S, Sotonyi P, et al. Minireview: Ghrelin and the regulation of energy balance–A hypothalamic perspective. Endocrinology. 2001;142:4163-4169.

38. Morash B, Li A, Murphy PR, et al. Leptin gene expression in the brain and pituitary gland. Endocrinology. 1999;140:5995-5998.

39. Bagnasco M, Kalra PS, Kalra SP. Ghrelin and leptin pulse discharge in fed and fasted rats. Endocrinology. 2002;143:726-729.

40. Beretta E, Dube MG, Kalra PS, Kalra SP. Long-term suppression of weight gain, adiposity, and serum insulin by central leptin gene therapy in prepubertal rats: Effects on serum ghrelin and appetite-regulating genes. Ped. Res. 2002;52:189-198.

41. Dube MG, Beretta E, Dhillon H, et al. Central leptin gene therapy blocks high fat diet-induced weight gain, hyperleptinemia and hyperinsulinemia: Effects on serum ghrelin levels. Diabetes. 2002;51:1729-1736.

42. Ueno N, Dube MG, Katz A, et al. Leptin inhibits ghrelin-induced obesity by two distinct central and peripheral mechanisms: Effects on adiponectin, 33rd Annual Society for Neuroscience Meeting, New Orleans, LA, November 2003.

43. Considine RV, Sinha MK, Heiman ML, et al. Serum immunoreactive-leptin concentrations in normal-weight and obese humans. N Engl J Med. 1996;334:292-295.

44. Pu S, Dube MG, Kalra PS, Kalra SP. Regulation of leptin secretion: Effects of aging on daily patterns of serum leptin and food consumption. Regul Pept. 2000; 92:107-111.

45. Dhillon H, Kalra SP, Prima V, et al. Central leptin gene therapy suppresses body weight gain, adiposity and serum insulin without affecting food consumption in normal rats: A long-term study. Regul Pept. 2001;99:69-77.

46. Kalra PS, Kalra SP. Obesity and metabolic syndrome: Long-term benefits of central leptin gene therapy. In: Prous, JR Ed. Drugs of Today. Barcelona, Spain: Prous Science, 2002; 38:745-757.

47. Kalra SP. Circumventing leptin resistance for weight control. Proc Natl Acad Sci. 2001;98:4279-4281.

48. Wise RA. Brain reward circuitry: Insights from unsensed incentives. Neuron. 2002;36:229-240.

49. Holderness CC, Brooks-Gunn J, Warren MP. Co-morbidity of eating disorders and substance abuse review of the literature. Int J Eat Disord. 1994;16:1-34.

50. Koob GF, Le Moal M. Drug addiction, dysregulation of reward, and allostasis. Neuropsychopharmacology. 2001;24:97-129.

51. Thiele TE, Marsh DJ, Ste Marie L, et al. Ethanol consumption and resistance are inversely related to neuropeptide Y levels. Nature. 1998;396:366-369.

52. Ehlers CL, Li TK, Lumeng L, et al. Neuropeptide Y levels in ethanol-naive alcohol-preferring and nonpreferring rats and in Wistar rats after ethanol exposure. Alcohol Clin Exp Res. 1998;22:1778-1782.

53. Hwang BH, Zhang JK, Ehlers CL, et al. Innate differences of neuropeptide Y (NPY) in hypothalamic nuclei and central nucleus of the amygdala between selectively bred rats with high and low alcohol preference. Alcohol Clin Exp Res. 1999;23:1023-1030.

54. Clark JT, Keaton AK, Sahu A, et al. Neuropeptide Y (NPY) levels in alcoholic and food restricted male rats: Implications for site selective function. Regul Pept. 1998;75-76:335-345.

55. Kelley SP, Nannini MA, Bratt AM, Hodge CW. Neuropeptide-Y in the paraventricular nucleus increases ethanol self-dministration. Peptides. 2001;22:515-522.

56. Woldbye DP, Ulrichsen J, Haugbol S, Bolwig TG. Ethanol withdrawal in rats is attenuated by intracerebroventricular administration of neuropeptide Y. Alcohol. 2002; 37:318-321.

57. Thiele TE, Koh MT, Pedrazzini T. Voluntary alcohol consumption is controlled via the neuropeptide Y Y1 receptor. J Neurosci. 2002;22:RC208.

58. Okubo T, Harada S. Polymorphism of the neuropeptide Y gene: An association study with alcohol withdrawal. Alcohol Clin Exp Res. 2001;25:59S-62S.

59. Fulton S, Woodside B, Shizgal P. Modulation of brain reward circuitry by leptin. Science. 2000;287:125-128.

60. Kiefer F, Jahn H, Kellner M, et al. Leptin as a possible modulator of craving for alcohol. Arch Gen Psychiatry. 2001;58:509-510.

61. Obradovic T, Meadows GG. Chronic ethanol consumption increases plasma leptin levels and alters leptin receptors in the hypothalamus and the perigonadal fat of C57BL/6 mice. Alcohol Clin Exp Res. 2002;26:255-262.

62. Fride E. Endocannabinoids in the central nervous system–an overview. Prostaglandins Leukot Essent Fatty Acids. 2002;66:221-233.

63. Williams CM, Kirkham TC. Reversal of delta 9-THC hyperphagia by SR141716 and naloxone but not dexfenfluramine. Pharmacol Biochem Behav. 2002;71:333-340.

64. Williams CM, Kirkham TC. Observational analysis of feeding induced by Delta 9-THC and anandamide. Physiol Behav. 2002;76:241-250.

65. Williams CM, Kirkham TC. Anadamide induces overeating: Mediation by central cannabinoid (CBI) receptors. Psychopharmacology.1999;143:315-317.

66. Di Marzo V, Goparaju SK, Wang L, et al. Leptin-regulated endocannabinoids are involved in maintaining food intake. Nature. 2001;410:822-825.

67. Kirkham TC, Williams CM, Fezza F, DiMarzo V. Endocannabinoid levels in rat limbic forebrain and hypothalamus in relation to fasting, feeding and satiation: Stimulation of eating by 2-arachidonoyl glycerol. Br J Pharmacol. 2002;136:550-557.

68. Jamshidi N, Taylor DA. Anadamide administration into the ventromedial hypothalamus stimulates appetite in rats. Br J Pharmacol. 2001;134:1151-1154.

69. Albanes D, Jones DY, Micozzi MS, Mattson ME. Associations between smoking and body weight in the US population: Analysis of NHANES II. Am J Public Health. 1987;77:439-444.

70. O'Hara P, Connett JE, Lee WW, et al. Early and late weight gain following smoking cessation in the Lung Health Study. Am J Epidemiol. 1998;148:821-830.

71. Li MD, Kane JK, Parker SL, et al. Nicotine administration enhances NPY expression in the rat hypothalamus. Brain Res. 2000;867:157-164.

72. Lupien JR, Bray GA. Nicotine increases thermogenesis in brown adipose tissue in rats. Pharmacol Biochem Behav. 1988;29:33-37.

73. Yoshida T, Sakane N, Umekawa T, et al. Nicotine induces uncoupling protein 1 in white adipose tissue of obese mice. Int J Obes Relat Metab Disord. 1999;23:570-575.

74. Hodge AM, Westerman RA, de Courten MP, et al. Is leptin sensitivity the link between smoking cessation and weight gain? Int J Obes Relat Metab Disord. 1997;21:50-53.

75. Li MD, Parker SL, Kane JK. Regulation of feeding-associated peptides and receptors by nicotine. Mol Neurobiol. 2000;22:143-165.

76. Kane JK, Parker SL, Matta SG, et al. Nicotine up-regulates expression of orexin and its receptors in rat brain. Endocrinology. 2000;141:3623-3629.

77. Kalra PS, Dube MG, Xu B, et al. Neuropeptide Y (NPY) Y1 receptor mRNA is upregulated in association with transient hyperphagia and body weight gain: Evidence for a hypothalamic site for concurrent development of leptin resistance. J Neuroendocrinol. 1998;10:43-49.

78. Kalra SP, Xu B, Dube MG, et al. Leptin and ciliary neurotropic factor (CNTF) inhibit fasting-induced suppression of luteinizing hormone release in rats: Role of neuropeptide Y. Neurosci Lett. 1998;240:45-49.

79. Morley JE, Levine AS, Yim GK, Lowy MT. Opioid modulation of appetite. Neurosci Biobehav Rev. 1983;7:281-305.

80. Levine AS, Billington CJ. Opioids. Are they regulators of feeding? Ann N Y Acad Sci. 1989;575:209-219.

81. Kalra PS, Norlin M, Kalra SP. Neuropeptide Y stimulates beta-endorphin release in the basal hypothalamus: Role of gonadal steroids. Brain Res. 1995;705:353-356.

82. Brugman S, Clegg DJ, Woods SC, Seeley RJ. Combined blockade of both micro- and kappa-opioid receptors prevents the acute orexigenic action of Agouti-related protein. Endocrinology. 2002;143:4265-4270.

83. Lambert PD, Wilding JP, al-Dokhayel AA, et al. The effect of central blockade of kappa-opioid receptors on neuropeptide Y-induced feeding in the rat. Brain Res. 1993;629:146-148.

Interaction of Satiety and Reward Response to Food Stimulation

G. Andrew James, PhD
Mark S. Gold, MD
Yijun Liu, PhD

SUMMARY. Obesity is among the most pressing health issues affecting developed countries. The etiology of obesity remains unclear despite its associated health risks and problems. We propose a framework for obesity modeled upon overeating as a substance dependence disorder arising from a combination of abnormal cognitive and neuroendocrine processes. While significant work has investigated the body's regulation of satiety signals, fewer studies have focused on the mechanisms by which these two seemingly disparate (cognitive and neuroendocrine) systems interact. Although emotional states have been shown to mediate reward processing, the implications for hunger mediating reward have not previously been addressed. We review the interaction between cen-

---

G. Andrew James, Mark S. Gold, and Yijun Liu are affiliated with the University of Florida College of Medicine, Departments of Psychiatry and Neuroscience, and McKnight Brain Institute, Gainesville, FL.

Address correspondence to: Yijun Liu, PhD, The University of Florida McKnight Brain Institute, Department of Psychiatry, 100 South Newell Drive, L4-100, Gainesville, FL 32610-0256.

The authors are grateful to Dr. A. G. He for assistance in MRI data acquisition. This work was supported in part by grant from National Institutes of Health (NS45518 and DA16221).

[Haworth co-indexing entry note]: "Interaction of Satiety and Reward Response to Food Stimulation." James, G. Andrew, Mark S. Gold, and Yijun Liu. Co-published simultaneously in *Journal of Addictive Diseases* (The Haworth Medical Press, an imprint of The Haworth Press, Inc.) Vol. 23, No. 3, 2004, pp. 23-37; and: *Eating Disorders, Overeating, and Pathological Attachment to Food: Independent or Addictive Disorders?* (ed: Mark S. Gold) The Haworth Medical Press, an imprint of The Haworth Press, Inc., 2004, pp. 23-37. Single or multiple copies of this article are available for a fee from The Haworth Document Delivery Service [1-800-HAWORTH, 9:00 a.m. - 5:00 p.m. (EST). E-mail address: docdelivery@haworthpress.com].

http://www.haworthpress.com/web/JAD
© 2004 by The Haworth Press, Inc. All rights reserved.
Digital Object Identifer: 10.1300/J069v23n03_03

23

tral satiety signals and reward responses to food stimuli and discuss the implications of this research for understanding the causes of obesity. *[Article copies available for a fee from The Haworth Document Delivery Service: 1-800-HAWORTH. E-mail address: <docdelivery@ haworthpress.com> Website: <http://www.HaworthPress.com> © 2004 by The Haworth Press, Inc. All rights reserved.]*

KEYWORDS. Neuroimaging, fMRI, obesity, overeating

INTRODUCTION

Obesity is a serious health condition reaching pandemic proportions. Recent surveys indicate that, in the United States, one-third of men and women aged 20 years or older are overweight [body mass index (BMI) > 25.0].[1] The percentage of clinically obese (BMI > 30.0) individuals in the US has nearly doubled in the past two decades.[2] Health problems linked to obesity are numerous and include stroke, heart disease, non-insulin dependent diabetes mellitus, osteoarthritis, and increased risk for developing cancer.[3,4] The number of deaths relating to obesity rivals those attributed to alcohol- and nicotine-use.[5] But while researchers agree that obesity is a disease warranting increased public awareness, its relationship to depression, personality disorders and addiction are not as strongly emphasized. The similarities between overeating and substance use disorders have been established[6,7] as have the co-morbid disorders most commonly associated with these illnesses. Recent functional brain imaging studies have suggested that obesity and the inability to control eating behaviors produce changes in neural activity patterns similar to those produced by substance use.[8,9] Given these similarities, newly discovered physiological messengers that modulate eating behavior (i.e., leptin and ghrelin) may mediate not only obesity but also alcoholism and other drug dependencies.

THEORETICAL CAUSES OF OBESITY

Numerous theories attempt to explain the causes of obesity. A popular biologic theory is that obesity develops from abnormal neuro-endocrine processes involved in the control of eating behavior and energy homeostasis. Most of these theories focus upon the hypothalamus, a principal component of the central nervous system for maintaining energy homeostasis.[10,11] An alteration in hypothalamic response to anorexigenic or orexigenic signals could result in a delayed central sensation of satiety. The consequent feeding behavior would gradually lead to obesity.

Conversely, the prototypical cognitive approach cites the social implications of food as reward (e.g., having to clean one's plate for dessert) and focuses upon our behavioral responses to food rewards.[12] While these disparate approaches may initially seem irreconcilable, the regulation of hunger and satiety most likely stems from interaction between endocrine and cognitive processes.[13] The purpose of this review is to elaborate upon psychobiological processes mediating hunger and satiety.

Overeating as a Substance Dependence Disorder

Constructing a model for overeating as an addiction is inherently difficult due to the ambiguous psychological and psychiatric definitions of addiction. We instead model overeating as a substance dependence disorder. The comparison is imperfect since the DSM-IV does not recognize food as a substance of abuse. Furthermore, we are all physiologically dependent upon food for survival, so one could facetiously argue that everyone suffers from tolerance and withdrawal to food (two of three specifiers necessary for a diagnosis of substance dependence). The remaining specifiers for substance dependence (e.g., greater consumption of the substance than planned, failed attempts to cut back on consumption, etc.) reflect the difficulties many obese individuals experience when attempting to reduce food intake. When the criteria for physiological dependence are disregarded, food adequately fits the model for substance dependence.

We contend that obesity may be considered a byproduct of substance dependence with food as the substance in question. Within this theoretical framework, cognitive-behavioral therapies typically reserved for substance dependence therapies may be applicable toward the treatment of obesity.[14] However, treatment is beyond the scope of this review; we instead wish to review prominent functional neuroimaging research on the reward system and their common implications for substance dependence and obesity. We will also review a novel functional MRI (fMRI) method for studying the neuro-hormonal mediation of hunger and satiety based on our previous work,[15,16] focusing on the hypothalamus and its associated signaling pathways in regulating eating behavior and body-weight. Our ultimate goal is to provide a feasible model for the interaction of the nervous and endocrine systems in regulating both substance use and eating behaviors.

RECENT METHODOLOGY DEVELOPMENT AND FINDINGS

Functional Neuroanatomy of Reward

Reward-system circuitry and the learning of reward contingencies have been topics of study for many years. Excellent reviews can be found concerning the role of neurotransmitters in establishing and mediating reward incidents[17-19] as well as the neuroanatomy and connectivity of reward circuits.[20-22] These reviews stress two main circuits for mediating reward behaviors: a fronto-amygdalar pathway reciprocally connecting the amygdala and prefrontal (orbito-, ventromedial-, and dorsolateral-) cortices and a limbic circuit integrating the amygdala with the hypothalamus and septal nuclei. A second limbic circuit, Papez circuit, integrates the hypothalamus with hippocampus and thalamus. The hypothalamus is at the junction between these two limbic circuits, with the hippocampal branch forming new memories while the amygdalar branch assigns value judgments to those memories.

The tight connectivity of the limbic circuits with phylogenically ancient structures such as the insular cortex suggests that the limbic system is mostly concerned with unconditionally rewarding stimuli such as food, water, and sex.[23,24] In contrast, the fronto-amygdalar circuit may be more focused upon conditionally rewarding stimuli, such as money or abstract concepts.[25] The distinction, if any, between the rewards these circuits mediate can best be teased apart with functional imaging. More than merely a means for corroborating anatomical findings, functional imaging techniques including positron emission tomography (PET) and fMRI allow the unique perspective of viewing brain circuitry in vivo.[15,26] The inherently global nature of these techniques allows for the analysis of the spatial and temporal extent to which these anatomic reward circuits are activated. Individual differences in brain response to different rewarding stimuli can be assessed, as well as how these reward systems are perturbed by long-term drug abuse.

Substance Dependence

Nowhere is the synthesis of biological and physiological reward mechanisms more prominent than in substance dependence literature.

Nicotine dependence, for example, can produce cue- and environment-dependent cravings so powerful that substance users will selectively pursue nicotine reinforcement over competing unconditional reinforcers.[27,28] Substance dependence is particularly relevant to the discussion of reward since dependent users will continue to pursue the substance in question despite punishing factors inherent to substance use (i.e., unsanitary environments, detrimental health effects) and from external sources (i.e., disapproval of family and peers, legal and economic consequences). Long-term substance use results in physiological changes in the responsiveness of reward circuitry to the substance of use.[29]

Cocaine dependence exemplifies these changes in the neural systems mediating reward. Bonson et al. monitored the neural activity of people with cocaine dependencies as they were exposed to cocaine-related cues and neutral cues.[30] The previous study on cocaine users demonstrated increased activation of the right dorsolateral prefrontal cortex, left lateral orbitofrontal cortex, and left ventrolateral amygdala in response to cocaine-related cues over neutral cues, with the activity of these regions positively correlating to the participants' self-reported degree of cocaine craving. Importantly, increased activity was not observed in areas not associated with reward, such as the paracentral cortex, posterior thalamus, globus pallidus and caudate nucleus, so the activation was specific to reward and not a global change in activity due to increased arousal.[31] The observed patterns of reward circuitry activity generalize to other forms of addiction; for example, nicotine-deprived smokers demonstrate increased activation of both limbic circuits (the amygdala, hippocampus, ventral tegmental area, and thalamus) in response to smoking-cues over nonsmoking-cues.[32] These previous studies emphasize that substances of abuse can alter both frontal and limbic responses.

It should come as no surprise that cues relating to substances of abuse activate the reward systems of individuals dependent upon those substances. But how does substance dependency affects the processing of non-substance rewards? Functional neuroimaging has shown activity of the limbic system and prefrontal cortices to vary with monetary gain or loss.[33] While patients with nicotine-dependencies and healthy control populations had comparable limbic activity in response to monetary awards, dopaminergic areas such as the striatum were activated to monetary rewards in smokers and nonmonetary rewards in nonsmokers.[34] One interpretation for these findings is that reward processing becomes anchored to the substance of dependence, and a given stimulus is rewarding only insofar as it can aid the subjects with addiction in obtaining the substance in question. However, it is possible that this decrease in activation is an inherent condition that predisposes a person toward obtaining concrete rewards such as drugs over abstract rewards. The causal nature of this relationship remains to be clarified with further research. Another interpretation of this study concerns the postulation proposed earlier that the fronto-amygdalar circuit deals with abstract, goal-oriented rewards whereas the limbic system focuses upon more basic rewards. Clearly, such an attribution is far more complex than previously stated if not patently false.

Emotional Modulation of Reward

The previously described studies pose the following question: does a pre-existing neurological condition predispose one toward substance dependence? While the answer to this question is beyond the scope of this review, aberrant responses to reinforcing stimuli have been observed in populations suffering from psychiatric disorders. It has recently been proposed that obsessive-compulsive disorder (OCD) is not merely an anxiety disorder but is also driven by disgust.[35] Neuroimaging studies support this theory with the finding that OCD and control populations express similar patterns of brain activity in response to threatening visual-stimuli designed to induce fear and anxiety, whereas the activity patterns differ between the two groups for disgust-inducing stimuli.[36] OCD patients viewing pictures of contaminated food had significant increases in insular activity (a region responsive to both gustatory stimuli and disgust) but significant decreases in medial prefrontal cortex activity relative to control populations. One can conclude that OCD patients found contamination-related stimuli more disgusting than did control subjects. These findings demonstrate an interaction between an individual's emotional state (in this case, disgust) and the valence of a stimulus. Although the causal nature of this relationship has not been formally established, emotion is most likely influencing reward processing in this instance since OCD is commonly considered an anxiety or affective disorder. Given the coterminous nature of the two limbic circuits, it is both feasible and probable that an affective disorder can alter the value judgments placed upon rewarding or punishing stimuli.

The Biochemical and Physiological Processes of Satiety

We have illustrated how psychiatric conditions such as addiction and OCD can influence the relative reward value of stimuli. The eating disorder literature lends more credence to this theory. The endocrine response to fasting and the biochemical means by which the body mediates hunger and satiety is addressed (see Kalra & Kalra: Overlapping and interactive pathways regulating appetite and craving, in this issue). But how do these neurochemical signaling pathways translate into behavior? What cognitive mechanisms influence reward processing so as to vary the reward value of food relative to other reinforcers as a function of the organism's satiety level? When and under what conditions does the interface between biochemical signaling and cognitive awareness occur?

Functional neuroimaging addresses these questions by monitoring the brain response to perturbations of the endocrine system. The fMRI technique of temporal clustering analysis (TCA) has been developed to identify when changes in brain activity occur throughout the course of a functional scan.[15] TCA operates by searching the time course of a scan, second by second, for significant fluctuations in brain activity. Once it is determined when changes in brain activity occur, further analysis can be conducted to evaluate how and where brain response changes for these durations. TCA has been applied to assess changes in brain response to glucose administration in healthy fasting volunteers. Brain activity was shown to significantly change around 9 minutes following glucose ingestion in normal weight subjects (Figure 1). After isolating the duration of enhanced brain activity, statistical parametric mapping revealed significant decreases in hypothalamic activity, with this activity correlated with plasma insulin levels.[9,15] Interestingly, in obese subjects, such changes in fMRI measurement was significantly delayed and attenuated.[16]

Perhaps more intriguing is that plasma insulin levels did not correlate with the decreases in hypothalamic activity in obese fasting volunteers,[9] while they did correlate in lean subjects. The lack of coordination between hypothalamic response and plasma insulin concentration conceivably translates into a delayed awareness of satiety. An inherent response latency of this nature could easily lead to a history of overeating and thus provide a neurobiological explanation for obesity.

Reward and Hunger

While this previous work lays the groundwork for a bottom-up approach combining biochemical and neuropsychological methods for studying brain-body modulation of hunger, other work has adopted a more cognitive approach. Morris and Dolan examined how one's hun-

FIGURE 1. Glucose-induced hypothalamic activity in lean and obese subjects. Spatial parametric mapping localized brain activity 7-14 minutes after glucose ingestion to the ventromedial hypothalamus.

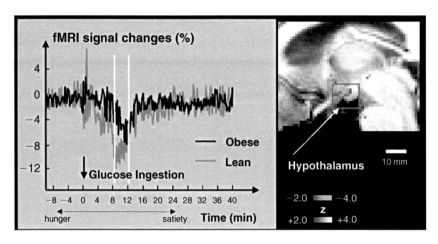

ger state can influence memory for food-related stimuli.[37] Fasting subjects had increased recognition for previously viewed food stimuli over sated subjects. While the activity of limbic and limbic associated structures (hypothalamus, insula, and nucleus accumbens) covaried positively with hunger ratings and left amygdalar activity covaried positively with recognition for food items, only orbitofrontal cortex activity covaried positively as a function of food and hunger state. Specifically, the right anterior orbitofrontal cortex was found to covary positively with recognition for all stimuli (food and non-food) irregardless of hunger state, whereas the right posterior orbitofrontal cortex only covaried positively for food stimuli during the hunger (and not sated) state. This finding is intriguing in that it suggests dissociable roles for the orbitofrontal cortex and the anterior region seeking reward for correctly recognizing previously viewed stimuli, but the posterior region responsive to more internal reward. The specter of differing neural correlates for abstract versus concrete rewards arises again, but such dissociation is tenuously supported at best in the absence of corroborating data.

A shortcoming for many hunger studies is that stimuli cause both valence and arousal. Failure to control for the arousing properties of presented stimuli can confound neuroimaging studies, as increased arousal could lead to an artifactual apparent increase in reward system activity.

To control for arousal effects, a fasting study has been performed incorporating visual stimuli from the International Affective Picture System (IAPS).[38] By comparing pictures of food (and food-related) items to pictures of animals and tools matched for valence and arousal (Figure 2), the effects of these two properties on neural reward circuits can be teased apart. A comparison of food items to non-food items (low valence, low arousal) resulted in activation of the insula, the prefrontal cortex, the amygdala, the thalamus, and especially the nucleus accumbens at the ventral basal ganglia in hungry but not sated subjects.[39] While these findings are indicative of brain activity specific to hunger, a comparison of food versus arousing animals (or even food-related tools to nonfood-related tools) is necessary to eliminate the confound from arousal.

FUTURE DIRECTIONS

As previously mentioned, an altered hypothalamic response to glucose ingestion may reflect the change in the central satiety signal that is associated with obesity and changes in the peripheral hormonal levels;[9] however, the relationship currently lacks causal directionality. Although a study of obese individuals using the fasting paradigm described above would determine how obese individuals react differently than non-obese individuals to rewarding food stimuli while discriminating for arousal effects, such a study still cannot elucidate whether changes in reward circuitry lead to obesity or are a result of obesity. It is important to reiterate that, while animal models would be ideal for finding a double-dissociation, functional imaging on clinical populations would be more beneficial for defining the causal relationship between biochemical changes in satiety and psychobiological changes in reward values caused by obesity and substance dependence. Following are our ongoing fMRI studies in three different directions.

Satiety in Prader-Willi Syndrome

A solution for this causality issue may lie in study of patients with Prader-Willi Syndrome (PWS), a neurogenetic multisystem disorder characterized by infantile hypotonia, mental retardation, short stature, hypogonadism, dysmorphic features, and hyperphagia with a high risk of obesity.[40] The behavioral symptoms in patients with PWS include compulsions toward binge eating and obesity, with typical onset just

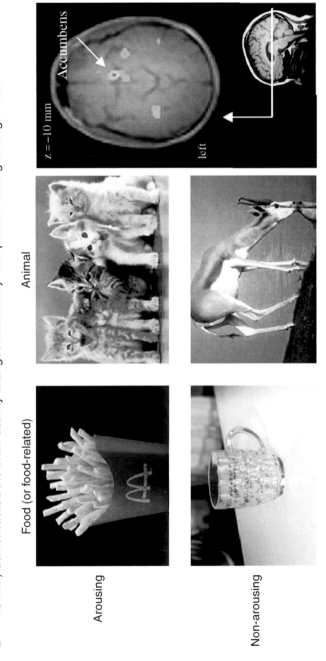

FIGURE 2. Arousing and non-arousing rewarding stimuli. A comparison of stimuli matched for valence and arousal (top row) allows for the identification of changes in reward processing with hunger. In contrast, a comparison of stimuli matched for valence but not arousal (columns) allows for the identification of neural changes due to arousal both independent (right column; animal) and dependent (left column; food) upon hunger state. The functional activation map at an axial brain section through the accumbens nucleus and the posterior orbitofrontal cortex (the Talairach coordinate z = −10 mm) demonstrated the brain activity changes induced by food pictures during a hunger state.

prior to puberty. An analysis of reward circuit activity using fMRI immediately following the onset of behavioral symptoms would clarify if hunger mediates reward response or vice versa. For example, a disruption of hypothalamic activity would suggest that an altered satiety response[41] eventually results in modulation of reward processing, whereas variations in reward circuit activity suggest a cognitive alteration in hypothalamic function. The running question of whether or not different reward circuits mediate abstract versus concrete rewards may well be answered by this study, as food rewards may be perceived with greater value in binge eaters.

Expression of Hunger or Fasting in Hypoglycemia Unawareness

Hypoglycemia unawareness (i.e., development of neuroglycopenia without appropriate prior awareness of autonomic warning symptoms) is a frequent and potentially dangerous syndrome and becomes the most important acute complication in type I diabetes after long-term intensive insulin treatment. Because hypoglycemia often occurs suddenly and unpredictably, patients with hypoglycemia unawareness cannot correct impending hypoglycemia (e.g., by eating food).[42] Therefore, the condition of hypoglycemia unawareness can be used to address the means by which healthy individuals are consciously aware of hunger and satiety.

Although hunger and fasting are terms typically used interchangeably, the distinction needs to be made that fasting is a quantifiable biological phenomenon whereas hunger is more akin to a mood or emotional state. While hunger is an emergent state arising from fasting, cognitive processes can undoubtedly influence one's perception of hunger, resulting in marked individual differences in hunger sensation. An analysis of hypoglycemia unawareness using our current fMRI paradigms can shed light upon how the hunger state develops from fasting and what emotional or reward processing factors attenuate that state. While the interactions between satiety, cognition, and reward processing are undoubtedly complex, careful investigation of these phenomena will certainly clarify the mechanisms by which these seemingly disparate processes interact.

Brain Modulation of Reward in Obese Tobacco Users

Finally, if hunger is viewed in the context as being an addiction, the question inevitably arises of how the neural mechanisms regulating satiety and those regulating addictive rewards interact. For example, the nicotine literature is ripe with studies citing weight gain among chronic smokers upon smoking cessation, with this potential weight gain acting as a deterrent (especially among women) against quitting.[43,44] The finding of elevated leptin levels among chronic smokers could link hunger to addiction.[45,46] A functional neuroimaging investigation into the neuroendocrine regulation of leptin among chronic smokers would have a two-fold purpose: not only would such a study further specify the mechanisms by which leptin may mediate satiety, but the potential of leptin for mediating signaling among reward circuitry would be assessed. Research into the direct interaction of hunger and reward circuitry is essential for pinning down the transitional boundaries between biology and psychology, with investigations of this nature shedding light upon the brain modulation of reward by emotion and obesity.

CONCLUSIONS

Redefining obesity as the product of a substance dependence disorder would alleviate the stigma associated with this illness while providing new directions for treating this growing epidemic. We acknowledge that the causal relationship between eating behaviors and the observed alterations in neurobiological reward circuitry remains to be established, most likely though the study of genetic conditions with accompanying eating disorders (i.e., Prader-Willi Syndrome). Although the DSM-IV does not recognize food as a substance of abuse, the converging neuroimaging, cognitive, and behavioral findings presented above suggest that food feasibly fits within the model of substance dependence. Such a framework would necessitate further study of biochemical messengers such as leptin and ghrelin, whose traditional roles in mediating hunger states may well transcend into modulating the relative reward of nonfood stimuli. Further research into these directions will grant us a truly comprehensive understanding of the complex neural and endocrine interactions driving our eating behaviors.

REFERENCES

1. Lyznicki JM, Young DC, Riggs JA, Davis RM. For the Council on Scientific Affairs. Obesity: Assessment and management in primary care. Am Fam Physician. 2001; 63:2185-96.

2. U.S. Department of Health and Human Services, Public Health Service. The Surgeon General's call to action to prevent and decrease overweight and obesity. Office of the Surgeon General. 2001; Available from: U.S. GPO, Washington.

3. Raman RP. Obesity and health risks. J Am Coll Nutr. 2002; 21:134S-9S.

4. Pi-Sunyer FX. The medical risks of obesity. Obesity Surgery. 2002; 12(1): 6S-11S.

5. Sturm R, Wells KB. Does obesity contribute as much to morbidity as poverty or smoking? Public Health. 2001; 115(3):229-35.

6. Jonas JM, Gold MS. Cocaine abuse and eating disorders. Lancet. 1986; 1:390-1.

7. Gold MS, Johnson CR, Stennie K. Eating Disorders. In: Lowinson JH, Ruiz P, Millman RB, Langrod JG, eds. Substance Abuse: A Comprehensive Textbook. 3rd ed. Philadelphia, PA: Lippincott, Williams and Wilkins, 1997:319-30.

8. Gautier JF, Chen K, Salbe AD, et al. Differential brain responses to satiation in obese and lean men. Diabetes. 2000; 49:838-46.

9. James GA, Guo W, Liu Y. Imaging in vivo brain-hormone interaction in the control of eating and obesity. Diabetes Technol Ther. 2001; 3:617-22.

10. Schwartz MW, Woods SC, Porte D Jr, et al. Central nervous system control of food intake. Nature. 2000; 404:661-71.

11. Woods SC, Seeley RJ. Understanding the physiology of obesity: Review of recent developments in obesity research. Int J Obes Relat Metab Disord. 2002; Suppl 4:S8-S10.

12. Shizgal P, Fulton S, Woodside B. Brain reward circuitry and the regulation of energy balance. Int J Obes Relat Metab Disord. 2001; 25: Suppl 5, S17-S21.

13. Saper CB, Chou TC, Elmquist JK. The need to feed: Homeostatic and hedonic control of eating. Neuron. 2002; 36:199-211.

14. Kadden RM. Behavioral and cognitive-behavioral treatments for alcoholism: Research opportunities. Addictive Behaviors. 2001; 26(4):489-507.

15. Liu Y, Gao JH, Liu HL, Fox PT. The temporal response of the brain after eating revealed by functional MRI. Nature. 2000; 405:1058-62.

16. Matsuda M, Liu Y, Mahankali S, et al. Altered hypothalamic response to oral glucose intake in obese humans. Diabetes. 1999; 48:1801-6.

17. Schultz W. Multiple reward signals in the brain. Nature Rev Neurosci. 2000; 1(3):199-207.

18. Schultz W. Getting formal with dopamine and reward. Neuron. 2002; 36: 241-63.

19. Tzschentke TM. Pharmacology and behavioral pharmacology of the meso-cortical dopamine system. Prog Neurobio. 2001; 63:241-320.

20. Breiter HC, Rosen BR. Functional magnetic resonance imaging of brain reward circuitry in the human. Ann N Y Acad Sci. 1999; 877:523-47.

21. Rolls ET. The orbitofrontal cortex and reward. Cerebral Cortex. 2000; 10: 284-94.

22. Baxter MG, Murray EA. The Amygdala and Reward. Nature Rev Neurosci. 2002; 3:563-73.

23. Denton D, Shade R, Zamarippa F, et al. Neuroimaging of genesis and satiation of thirst and an interoceptor-driven theory of origins of primary consciousness. Proc Natl Acad Sci USA. 1999; 96:5304-9.

24. Augustine JR. Circuitry and functional aspects of the insular lobe in primates including humans. Brain Res Rev. 1996; 22:229-44.

25. O'Doherty J, Kringelbach ML, Rolls ET, et al. Abstract reward and punishment representations in the human orbitofrontal cortex. Nature Neurosci. 2001;4:95-102.

26. Tataranni PA, Gautier JF, Chen K, et al. Neuroanatomical correlates of hunger and satiation in humans using positron emission tomography. Proc Natl Acad Sci USA. 1999; 96:4569-74.

27. Caggiula AR, Donny EC, White AR, et al. Cue dependency of nicotine self-administration and smoking. Pharmacology, Biochemistry and Behavior. 2001; 70:515-30.

28. Schroeder BE, Binzak JM, Kelly AE. A common profile of prefrontal cortical activation following exposure to nicotine- or chocolate-associated contextual cues. Neuroscience. 2001; 105:535-45.

29. Goldstein RZ, Volkow ND. Drug addiction and its underlying neurobiological basis: neuroimaging evidence for the involvement of the frontal cortex. Am J Psychiatry. 2002; 129:1642-52.

30. Bonson KR, Grant SJ, Contoreggi CS, et al. Neural systems and cue-induced cocaine craving. Neuropsychopharmacology. 2002; 26:376-86.

31. Lang PJ, Bradley MM, Fitzsimmons JR, et al. Emotional arousal and activation of the visual cortex: An fMRI analysis. Psychophysiology. 1998; 35:199-210.

32. Due DL, Huettel SA, Hall WG, Rubin DC. Activation in mesolimbic and visuospatial neural circuits elicited by smoking cues: Evidence from functional magnetic resonance imaging. Am J Psychiatry. 2002; 159:954-60.

33. Elliot R, Friston KJ, Dolan RJ. Dissociable neural responses in human reward systems. J Neurosci. 2000; 20:6159-65.

34. Martin-Sölch C, Magyar S, Künig G, et al. Changes in brain activation associated with reward processing in smokers and nonsmokers: A positron emission tomography study. Exp Brain Res. 2001; 139:278-86.

35. Stein DJ, Liu Y, Shapira NA, Goodman WK. The psychobiology of obsessive-compulsive disorder: How important is the role of disgust? Curr Psychiatry Rep. 2001; 3:281-7.

36. Shapira NA, Liu Y, He AG. Brain activation by disgust-inducing pictures in obsessive-compulsive disorder. Bio Psychiatry. 2003; 54:751-6.

37. Morris JS, Dolan RJ. Involvement of human amygdala and orbitofrontal cortex in hunger-enhanced memory for food stimuli. J Neurosci. 2001; 21:5304-10.

38. Lang PJ, Bradley MM, Cuthbert BN. International affective picture system (IAPS): Instruction Manual and Affective Ratings. Technical Report A-5. 2001; The Center for Research in Psychophysiology, University of Florida. Gainesville, FL.

39. James GA, He AG, Miller AW, et al. MRI of hunger and insula activation during a fasting paradigm. Proceedings of International Society for Magnetic Resonance in Medicine. 2002; 10:817.

40. Clarke DJ, Boer H, Whittington H, et al. Prader-Willi syndrome, compulsive and ritualistic behaviors: The first population-based survey. Br J Psychiatry. 2002; 180:358-62.

41. Shapira NA, Lessig MC, Liu Y, et al. Neuroanatomical correlates of satiation and hunger in adults with Prader-Willi Syndrome: A study using fMRI. Abstract for the 17th Annual PWSA Scientific Conference 2002, Salt Lake City, CO.

42. Bolli GB. Prevention and treatment of hypoglycaemia unawareness in type 1 diabetes mellitus. Acta Diabetol. 1998; 35(4):183-93.

43. Pomerleau CS, Zucker AN, Stewart AJ. Characterizing concerns about post-cessation weight gain: Results from a national survey of women smokers. Nicotine Tob Res. 2001; 3:51-60.

44. Kennedy DT, Giles JT, Chang ZG, et al. Results of a smoking cessation clinic in community pharmacy practice. J Am Pharm Assoc (Wash). 2002; 42(1):51-6.

45. Oeser A, Goffaux J, Snead W, Carlson MG. Plasma leptin concentrations and lipid profiles during nicotine abstinence. Am J Med Sci. 1999; 318:152-7.

46. Perkins KA, Fonte C. Effects of smoking status and smoking cessation on leptin levels. Nicotine Tob Res. 2002; 4:459-66.

Similarity Between Obesity and Drug Addiction as Assessed by Neurofunctional Imaging: A Concept Review

Gene-Jack Wang, MD
Nora D. Volkow, MD
Panayotis K. Thanos, PhD
Joanna S. Fowler, PhD

SUMMARY. Overeating in obese individuals shares similarities with the loss of control and compulsive drug taking behavior observed in drug-addicted subjects. The mechanism of these behaviors is not well understood. Our prior studies with positron emission tomography (PET)

Gene-Jack Wang, Nora D. Volkow, Panayotis K. Thanos, and Joanna S. Fowler are all affiliated with the Medical and Chemistry Departments, Brookhaven National Laboratory, Upton, NY 11973 USA.

Currently Nora D. Volkow is affiliated with NIH/NIDA, Bethesda, MD 20892-9581.

Address correspondence to: Gene-Jack Wang, MD, Medical Department, Brookhaven National Laboratory, Upton, NY 11973 USA (E-mail: gjwang@bnl. gov).

This study was supported in part by grants from the U.S. Department of Energy (OBER), the National Institute on Drug Abuse (DA06891-06) and National Institute on Alcoholism and Alcohol Abuse (AA/ODO9481-04). The authors also thank the scientific and technical staffs at the Brookhaven Center for Imaging and Neurosciences for their support of these research studies as well as the individuals who volunteered for these studies.

[Haworth co-indexing entry note]: "Similarity Between Obesity and Drug Addiction as Assessed by Neurofunctional Imaging: A Concept Review." Wang, Gene-Jack et al. Co-published simultaneously in *Journal of Addictive Diseases* (The Haworth Medical Press, an imprint of The Haworth Press, Inc.) Vol. 23, No. 3, 2004, pp. 39-53; and: *Eating Disorders, Overeating, and Pathological Attachment to Food: Independent or Addictive Disorders?* (ed: Mark S. Gold) The Haworth Medical Press, an imprint of The Haworth Press, Inc., 2004, pp. 39-53. Single or multiple copies of this article are available for a fee from The Haworth Document Delivery Service [1-800-HAWORTH, 9:00 a.m. - 5:00 p.m. (EST). E-mail address: docdelivery@ haworthpress.com].

http://www.haworthpress.com/web/JAD
Digital Object Identifer: 10.1300/J069v23n03_04

39

in drug-addicted subjects documented reductions in striatal dopamine (DA) D2 receptors. In pathologically obese subjects, we found reductions in striatal DA D2 receptors similar to that in drug-addicted subjects. Moreover, DA D2 receptor levels were found to have an inverse relationship to the body mass index of the obese subjects. We postulated that decreased levels of DA D2 receptors predisposed subjects to search for reinforcers; in the case of drug-addicted subjects for the drug and in the case of the obese subjects for food as a means to temporarily compensate for a decreased sensitivity of DA D2 regulated reward circuits. Understanding the mechanism in food intake will help to suggest strategies for the treatment of obesity. *[Article copies available for a fee from The Haworth Document Delivery Service: 1-800-HAWORTH. E-mail address: <docdelivery@haworthpress.com> Website: <http://www.HaworthPress.com>]*

KEYWORDS. Dopamine receptor, drug abuse, obesity, positron emission tomography, somatosensory cortex

INTRODUCTION

Obesity is a complex disease of appetite regulation and energy metabolism that is controlled by many factors.[1] It can result from several possible genetic and environmental interactions[2] some of which may entail a more direct genetic association (i.e., a genetically regulated response to sweet food which is perceived as reinforcing)[3] or alternatively an indirect association that makes the individual genetically more susceptible to environmental stressors that will then favor food consumption.[4]

Among the genetic factors, there are neuromodulators (e.g., leptin),[5] and multiple neurotransmitter systems involved with the reinforcing properties of food (i.e., GABA, dopamine, opioids, serotonin). These neurotransmitters also play an important role in feeding behavior and satiation.[6] There is a large amount of evidence to suggest that dopamine (DA) may be one of the neurotransmitters linking the genetic and environmental factors that contribute to obesity.[7] Behavioral studies on rodents indicate that DA D2 receptor antagonists can enhance meal size and duration of feeding.[8] Similarly, long-term administration of DA D2 receptor antagonists increases feeding and body weight in female rats.[9] In clinical studies, patients treated with typical and atypical antipsychotic medications, which block DA D2 receptors, show significant weight gain.[10,11] Dopaminergic agonists (e.g., amphetamine, cocaine, methylphenidate) that increase brain dopamine concentration have anorexigenic effects.[12]

Many obesity researchers focus on how the body's fuel and fat levels control appetite. But as binge eaters know, habits and desires often override metabolic need, which share some of the characteristics of drug using behavior in drug-addicted subjects. The present article discusses the role of DA in drug abuse and its involvement in the mechanism of obesity.

BRAIN DA AND ADDICTIVE BEHAVIORS

The role of DA in addiction (loss of control and compulsive drug intake) is poorly understood. A plethora of studies have reported over the years the role of dopamine and its receptors on alcohol and drug abuse. One example is the role of DA on cocaine addiction, which is considered to be one of the most reinforcing of the abused drugs. Animal studies have shown that the ability of cocaine to block the dopamine transporters appears to be crucial for its reinforcing effects. In humans, the reinforcing effects of cocaine used intravenously or smoked can lead to rapid escalation of drug intake and compulsive drug administration. Animal studies indicate that DA D2 receptor levels mediate reinforcing responses to drugs of abuse. We have shown that overexpression of DA D2 receptors in the nucleus accumbens, which is the brain region associated with the reinforcing effects of drugs of abuse, in animals previously trained to self-administer alcohol resulted in a marked reduction in alcohol intake that returned to baseline levels as the DA D2 receptors decreased to their prior levels.[13,14]

While the studies on the effects of DA D2 receptor antagonists on the reinforcing effects of psychostimulants in humans have not been as conclusive as those in laboratory animals, they have shown a decrease in the subjective ratings of pleasant sensations and of the craving induced by cocaine.[15] The lower efficacy of DA D2 receptor antagonists reported in studies may reflect the fact that the doses used were lower than those used in laboratory animals and resulted in incomplete DA D2 receptor blockade.

USE OF IN VIVO IMAGING TO STUDY DRUG ADDICTION

Positron Emission Tomography (PET) is a medical imaging technology that uses radioactive positron-emitting atoms (i.e., carbon-11 and fluorine-18) to label and measure the concentration and movement of positron labeled compounds in living tissue. Positron emitter labeled radiotracers are used to label proteins that are of physiological relevance (i.e., receptors, transporters and enzymes) in the human brain. The measurement of DA D2 receptor using PET and [11C]raclopride has been used to assess neuropsychiatric disorders, substance abuse and aging (reviewed,[16]). Since [11C]raclopride is sensitive to endogenous DA concentration and its binding is reproducible,[17] it can also be used to measure relative changes in DA concentration secondary to pharmacological interventions. Methylphenidate is a cocaine-like psychostimulant that increases extracellular DA by blocking DA transporters. Methylphenidate-induced changes in [11C]raclopride striatal binding are interpreted as reflecting changes induced by DA occupancy of D2 receptors secondary to the changes in DA synaptic concentration.[17] The measure has been used as an indication of the responsivity of the DA system to pharmacological challenge. This strategy allowed us to evaluate the relationship between DA changes as assessed by the levels of DA D2 receptors occupancy and subjective perception of pleasure or euphoric "high," which is associated with rewarding effects of the drug.[18] We found the intensity of the "high" induced by methylphenidate was significantly correlated with the levels of released DA. The subjects who reported the most intense "high" were those who have the greatest increases of DA release. It appears that DA and DA D2 receptors play an important role in the reinforcing response to psychostimulants.

Even though the reinforcing effects of cocaine may involve the initial drug taking behavior, others factors might also contribute to the compulsive drug taking and the loss of control in addicts. Repeated cocaine self-administration often continues (because of acute tolerance to the pleasurable response) and sometimes, despite the presence of an aversive drug reaction.[19,20] Acute tolerance to cocaine can occur in recreational levels of cocaine consumption. This neurochemical response to cocaine is primarily caused by direct pharmacological effects of the drug rather than by the conditioning to external environmental cues.[21] Chronic administration of cocaine significantly impacts the brain DA system.[22] In fact, our prior [11C]raclopride-PET studies in drug-addicted subjects (cocaine,[23] methamphetamine,[24] alcoholics,[25] and heroin[26]) showed significant DA D2 receptor reductions in striatum (Figure 1). It has been hypothesized that compulsive disorders such as drug addiction, gambling and sex reflect a "Reward Deficiency Syndrome,"[27] that is speculated to be due in part to a reduction in DA D2 receptors.

FIGURE 1. Group average images of [^{11}C]raclopride (distribution volume ratio) PET images for 15 methamphetamine users (9 women and 6 men, age range 21-46 years, mean 32 ± 7 years old), their control subjects (6 women and 14 men, age range 21-43 years, mean age 31 ± 7 years old), 10 obese subjects (5 women and 5 men, mean 39 ± 7 years old, age range 26-54) and their control subjects (3 women and 7 men, age range 25-45 years, mean 37.5 ± 5.9 years old) at the level of the striatum. The images are scaled with respect to the maximum absolute value obtained on average image of the control subjects and presented using the gray scale where white represents the highest value and black represents the lowest value. Methamphetamine users and obese subjects have significantly lower measures of striatal dopamine D2 receptor availability than control subjects. Modified from references 24 and 59.

[^{11}C]Raclopride

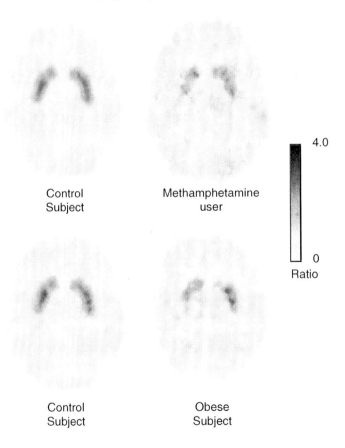

THE INVOLVEMENT OF BRAIN DA IN FOOD INTAKE

DA release seems to have a site-specific action on the regulation of food intake. In the nucleus accumbens, DA release has been generally associated with the reinforcing effects of food.[28] In the hypothalamus, DA release is associated with the duration of meal consumption, which is a factor in determining feeding pattern. Hence, DA is required to initiate each meal and is associated with the quantity and duration of a meal.[29] DA acting locally within the hypothalamus acts as a potent inhibitor of feeding in the perifornical area, ventromedial hypothalamus, and arcuate nucleus. In addition, DA is a potent inhibitor of hypothalamic neuropeptide Y (NPY, a potent stimulator of food intake) expression and activity and a stimulator of arcuate proopiomelanocortin (POMC) expression.[30,31] These hypothalamic influences may contribute to DA's ability to reduce food consumption and hyperphagia. Leptin, insulin, and other peripheral peptides and steroid hormones modulate the synthesis and release of DA.[32] It appears that DA is associated with both short-term (individual meals) and long-term (hunger) regulation of food intake.[33]

DA regulates food intake[34] via the meso-limbic circuitry of the brain apparently by modulating appetitive motivational processes.[35-37] There are also projections from the nucleus accumbens to the hypothalamus that directly regulate feeding.[38] The dopaminergic reward pathways of the brain are critical for survival since they help influence the fundamental drive for eating. Recent work has shown that DA systems are necessary for wanting incentives, which is a distinct component of motivation and reinforcement.[36,39] It is one of the natural reinforcing mechanisms that motivates an animal to perform and seek a given behavior. However, unnatural rewards such as drugs of abuse (i.e., cocaine, alcohol, nicotine), also release DA.[27] Furthermore, because most of the drugs abused by humans lead to increased DA concentration in the nucleus accumbens, this has been suggested as being a common mechanism for reinforcement.[19]

THE DOPAMINE'S ROLE IN THE MOTIVATION FOR FOOD INTAKE

Though the effects of DA in the nucleus accumbens are the ones traditionally implicated in motivation for food,[40] a study in DA deficient knockout mice provided clear evidence of the relevance of the dorsal striatum in the motivation for food consumption. Without intervention, these DA deficient mice die because of lack of food consumption, however, treatment with DA in the dorsal striatum, but not in the nucleus accumbens, restored feeding.[41] Interestingly in these animals rescuing DA in the nucleus accumbens restored the ability of the mice to choose between a palatable and a non-palatable solution but did not prevent them from dying due to inadequate caloric consumption. The latter study points to two separate processes regulating food intake; one to maintain the caloric requirements necessary for survival that implicates the dorsal striatum and another one that relates to the motivation properties of food (palatability) that implicates the nucleus accumbens.

To assess the involvement of DA in the dorsal striatum in the non-hedonic motivation for food intake in human subjects, we evaluated changes in extracellular DA in striatum in response to food stimulation (visual, olfactory, and gustatory display of food in food deprived subjects) after placebo and after methylphenidate.[41] In this study, methylphenidate was given as a strategy to amplify DA signals. Neither the neutral stimuli (with or without 20 mg of oral methylphenidate) nor the food stimuli when given with placebo increased DA or increased the desire for food. However, the food stimuli when given with methylphenidate increased both extracellular dopamine and the desire for food. We found that changes in extracellular dopamine in striatum in response to food stimulation were significant in dorsal but not in ventral striatum and were significantly correlated with the increases in self-reports of hunger and desire for food. Such a relationship was not observed for the ventral striatum where the nucleus accumbens is located. Our results showing an effect in the dorsal but not in the ventral striatum is likely to reflect the fact that the food stimulation to the subjects was not rewarding, i.e., in this study subjects were not permitted to consume the food.

THE ROLE OF BRAIN DOPAMINE IN OBESITY

DA plays a role in pathological feeding behavior, since low levels of DA may interfere with the drive and motivation to eat. Binge eating (Bulimia Nervosa), which occurs in about 30% of obese subjects attending weight control programs, is characterized by episodes of eating objectively large amounts of food and with feelings of loss of control.[42] Obese binge eaters consume significantly more calories than obese non-binge eaters when asked to eat as much as they wanted or simply to eat normally.[43,44] Obese binge eaters have high relapse rates during weight control programs and experience their disorder for long periods of time. A high prevalence of binge eating disorder (30-80%) was reported among the morbidly obese subjects who have undergone bariatric surgery.[45-49] The eating disturbances persist (6-26%) in many of the same patients after surgery and are correlated with weight regain.[45,47,49] The obese binge eaters lose less excess body weight than obese non-binge eaters after the surgery.[49]

Bulimic nervosa patients have been found to have normal DA metabolite levels. In contrast, high frequency binge eaters have reduced cerebrospinal fluid DA levels.[50] Decreased DA metabolite plasma levels have been found, but they are not associated with symptomatology of binge eating disorder.[51] To this day, it is difficult to determine whether a trait disturbance on the dopaminergic system plays a role in the etiology of binge eating disorder.

There is better evidence for the causal role of DA in obesity. Human studies have shown a higher prevalence of the Taq I A allele for the DA D2 receptors in obese subjects.[52] Though not replicated by all studies,[53] the Taq 1 A allele has been linked with lower levels of DA D2 receptors.[54] Variants of the human obesity (*ob*) gene and the DA D2 receptor gene have been examined in relationship to obesity. These two polymorphisms together account for about 20% of the variance in BMI, particularly in younger women.[55] The association of the Taq 1 A allele with reduced number of DA D2 receptor levels suggests that obese individuals with the A1 allele may use food to increase DA stimulation to a more desirable level.[56] This is consistent with the finding in binge eaters with frequent binge episodes who are reported to have low DA metabolite concentrations in cerebrospinal fluid.[51] These results indicate that low DA brain activity (either due to decreased DA release or to decreased stimulation of postsynaptic DA receptors) may be associated with dysfunctional eating patterns. The DA system has also been targeted for therapy of obesity since DA agonists have anorexigenic effects[57] whereas drugs that block DA D2 receptors increase appetite and result in weight gain.[58]

USE OF PET IMAGING TECHNOLOGY TO STUDY OBESITY

Compulsive overeating in obese subjects shares many of the same characteristics as drug addiction. Using a PET scanner with a re-designed bed to support heavy weight, we have shown a significant reduction in DA D2 receptor availability in obese subjects (Figure 1).[59] These subjects have body mass indexes (BMI: weight in kilograms divided by the square of height in meters) between 42 and 60 (mean 51.2 ± 4.8 kg/ m^2, body weight: 274-416 lb). These subjects do not have current or past psychiatric and/or neurological disease, hypertension, diabetes, and medical conditions that may alter cerebral functioning. Interestingly, in the obese subjects, but not in the controls, the DA D2 receptors were significantly associated with their BMI (Figure 2).[59] It is possible that in obese subjects, DA D2 receptors may play a greater role in regulating eating behavior than in control subjects. The results could also be interpreted to suggest that DA D2 receptors are not involved in modulating body weight per se but rather may regulate compulsiveness in the pathological eaters. This would imply that the role of the DA D2 receptors is not to enable obesity but if the pertinent genetic or environmental variables that predispose to obesity are present, then it will favor a more severe presentation. The obese subjects share in common with drug addicts the inability to refrain from using the reinforcer and its compulsive administration. Thus DA D2 decrements are unlikely to be specific for any one of these compulsive behavioral disorders including obesity and may relate to vulnerability for addictive behaviors.

DRUG PREFERENCES AND COMPULSIVE OVEREATING

One of the challenging questions regarding the neurobiological mechanism(s) underlying these disorders is why some subjects abuse drugs while others do not. We investigated this problem in non-drug abusing individuals in whom we measured DA D2 receptor levels and assessed their response (pleasant or unpleasant) to a challenge dose of the stimulant drug, methylphenidate given intravenously. We found that subjects who reported the methylphenidate as pleasant had lower DA D2 receptor levels.[60] Those who reported methylphenidate as unpleasant had higher DA D2 receptor levels. A replicate study documented that the levels of DA D2 receptors predicted how much subjects liked the effects of methylphenidate.[61] However, vulnerability to drug abuse could not be explained solely on the differences in DA D2 receptor availability since none of these subjects suffered from addiction even though they have very low DA D2 receptor levels. This indicates that while DA D2 receptors may contribute to vulnerability by themselves they are not sufficient to lead to addiction. Further work is neces-

FIGURE 2. Linear regression between dopamine receptor availability (Bmax/Kd) and body mass index (BMI: kg/m^2) in obese and control subjects. Modified from reference 59.

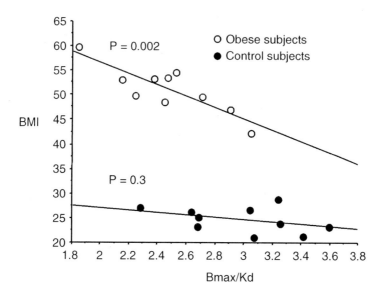

sary to assess if DA D2 receptors also modulate the "liking" responses to food to determine if low DA D2 levels may also be associated with a higher vulnerability for compulsive eating behaviors.

SENSORY PROCESSING OF THE FOOD AND OBESITY

What makes obese subjects different from drug addicts? Would obese subjects have an enhanced sensitivity in the brain regions involved with sensory processing of the food? Signals that affect food intake originate from internal sources that directly regulate food intake (i.e., hunger, satiety) and those that regulate emotional responses (i.e., to stress, boredom) as well as from the environmental sources (e.g., food availability, food related cues, alternative reinforcers).[62] Disruption in the sensitivity of the brain to these sources could lead to obesity from excess eating. Irrespective of the source, a particularly relevant variable in the regulation of food intake is the sensory appeal that the food conveys to the subject. Thus, we questioned whether obese subjects would have an enhanced sensitivity in the brain regions involved in sensory processing of the food associated with eating. We compared brain metabolism of obese subjects with lean control subjects using PET and 2-deoxy-2[^{18}F]fluoro-D-glucose (FDG), an analog of glucose, which has been served as an indicator of brain function. This method has been used to assess cerebral dysfunction in neurological and psychiatric disorders.[63] The brain metabolic images were analyzed using statistical parameter map (SPM), which showed that obese subjects had significantly greater glucose metabolism in the vicinity of the post-central gyrus in the left and right parietal cortex (Brodmann's areas 1).[64] This area of the parietal cortex is where the somatosensory maps of the mouth, lips, and tongue are located and is an area involved with taste perception (Figure 2).[65] The enhanced activation of these parietal regions is consistent with an enhanced sensitivity to food palatability (i.e., consistency, taste) in obese subjects. The enhanced activation in somatic parietal areas for mouth, tongue and lips in obese subjects suggests that enhanced sensitivity in regions involved in the sensory processing of food may make food more rewarding and may be one of the variables contributing to excess food consumption in these obese individuals.

MODULATION OF SENSORY PROCESSING OF THE FOOD IN OBESE INDIVIDUALS

Because foods with high palatability tend to have high energy content but are not satiating (fatty foods) in contrast to foods with low energy density that are more satiating but less palatable,[66] enhanced sensitivity to food palatability could lead to food over-consumption and obesity. Palatability increases food intake through a positive-feedback reward mechanism that involves the opioid and GABA/benzodiazepine systems.[67,68] Thus, interventions that include the use of pharmacological treatments known to decrease palatability (i.e., opioid receptor antagonist)[69] in association with behavioral therapies to reduce the likeness of food with high energy content may prove beneficial in reverting the enhanced sensitivity of the somatosensory areas processing food palatability and reducing food intake in obese subjects.

CONCLUSION

Though obesity is the product of many interacting variables, there is mounting evidence that the motivation and reward circuits regulated by

DA play a role. Our PET studies show obese individuals have significantly lower DA D2 receptor levels, which is similar to findings from PET studies in drug-addicted subjects. Lower DA D2 receptors in obese individuals would make them less sensitivity to reward stimuli, which in turn would make them more vulnerable to food intake as a means to temporarily compensate for this deficit. In addition, obese individuals show an enhanced activity of brain regions that process food palatability, which is likely to increase the rewarding properties of food and could account for the powerful salience that food has in obese individuals. The results from these studies have implications for the treatment of obesity since they would suggest that strategies aimed at improving DA function might be beneficial in the treatment and prevention of obesity.

REFERENCE

1. Serdula MK, Mokdad AH, Williamson DF, et al. Prevalence of attempting weight loss and strategies for controlling weight. JAMA 1999; 282:1353-1358.

2. Hill JO, Peters JC. Environmental contributions to the obesity epidemic. Science 1998; 280:1371-1374.

3. Smith GP, Schneider LH. Relationships between mesolimbic dopamine function and eating behavior. Ann N Y Acad Sci 1988; 537:254-261.

4. Greeno CG, Wing RR. Stress-induced eating. Psychol Bull 1994;115:444-464.

5. Bray GA, Tartaglia LA. Medicinal strategies in the treatment of obesity. Nature 2000; 404:672-677.

6. Schwartz MW, Woods SC, Porte D Jr, et al. Central nervous system control of food intake. Nature 2000; 404:661-671.

7. Blum K, Braverman ER, Holder JM, et al. Reward deficiency syndrome: a biogenetic model for the diagnosis and treatment of impulsive, addictive, and compulsive behaviors. J Psychoactive Drugs 2000;32 Suppl:1-112.

8. Clifton PG, Rusk IN, Cooper SJ. Effects of dopamine D1 and dopamine D2 antagonists on the free feeding and drinking patterns of rats. Behav Neurosci 1991; 105:272-281.

9. Baptista T, Parada M, Hernandez L. Long term administration of some antipsychotic drugs increases body weight and feeding in rats. Are D2 dopamine receptors involved? Pharmacol Biochem Behav 1987;27:399-405.

10. Allison DB, Casey DE. Antipsychotic-induced weight gain: a review of the literature. J Clin Psychiatry 2001;62 Suppl 7:22-31.

11. Wetterling T. Bodyweight gain with atypical antipsychotics. A comparative review. Drug Saf 2001;24:59-73.

12. Scislowski PW, Tozzo E, Zhang Y, et al. Biochemical mechanisms responsible for the attenuation of diabetic and obese conditions in ob/ob mice treated with dopaminergic agonists. Int J Obes Relat Metab Disord 1999;23:425-431.

13. Thanos PK, Volkow ND, Freimuth P, et al. Overexpression of dopamine D2 receptors reduces alcohol self-administration. J Neurochem 2001;78:1094-103.

14. Thanos PK, Taintor N, Hitzemann R, et al. The effect on ethanol drinking preference of D2 upregulation in the Nucleus Accumbens of the alcohol Preferring (P) and Non Preferring (NP) rats. Alcohol Clin Exp Res 2001;25 Suppl:56A.

15. Berger SP, Hall S, Mickalian JD, et al. Haloperidol antagonism of cue-elicited cocaine craving. Lancet 1996;347:504-508.

16. Farde L. The advantage of using positron emission tomography in drug research. Trends Neurosci 1996;19: 211-214.

17. Volkow ND, Wang G-J, Fowler JS, et al. Imaging endogenous dopamine competition with [^{11}C]Raclopride in the human brain. Synapse 1994;16: 255-262.

18. Volkow ND, Wang G-J, Fowler JS, et al. Reinforcing effects of psychostimulants in humans are associated with increases in brain dopamine and occupancy of D2 receptors. J Pharmacol Exp Ther 1999;291:409-415.

19. Fischman MW, Schuster CR, Javaid J, et al. Acute tolerance development to the cardiovascular and subjective effects of cocaine. J Pharmacol Exp Ther 1985;235: 677-682.

20. Koob GF, Bloom FE. Cellular and molecular mechanisms of drug dependence. Science 1988;242:715-723.

21. Bradberry CW. Acute and chronic dopamine dynamics in a nonhuman primate model of recreational cocaine use. J Neurosci 2000;20:7109-7115.

22. Moore RJ, Vinsant SL, Nader MA, et al. Effect of cocaine self-administration on dopamine D2 receptors in rhesus monkeys. Synapse 1998;30:88-96.

23. Volkow ND, Fowler JS, Wang G-J, et al. Decreased dopamine D2 receptor availability is associated with reduced frontal metabolism in cocaine abusers. Synapse 1993;14:169-177.

24. Volkow ND, Chang L, Wang G-J, et al. Decreased brain dopamine D2 receptors in methamphetamine abusers: association with metabolism in orbitofrontal cortex. Am J Psychiatry 2001;158:2015-2021.

25. Volkow ND, Wang G-J, Fowler JS, et al. Decreases in dopamine receptors but not in dopamine transporters in alcoholics. Alcohol Clin Exp Res 1996;20:1594-1598.

26. Wang G-J, Volkow ND, Fowler JS, et al. Dopamine D2 receptors availability in opiate-dependent subjects before and after naloxone-precipitated withdrawal. Neuropsychopharmacology 1997;16:174-182.

27. Blum K, Cull JG, Braverman ER, et al. Reward deficiency syndrome. American Scientist 1996;84:132-145.

28. Salamone JD, Cousins MS, Snyder BJ. Behavioral functions of nucleus accumbens dopamine: empirical and conceptual problems with the anhedonia hypothesis. Neurosci Biobehav Rev 1997;21:341-359.

29. Meguid MM, Fetissov SO, Varma M, et al. Hypothalamic dopamine and serotonin in the regulation of food intake. Nutrition 2000;16:843-857.

30. Tong Y, Pelletier G. Role of dopamine in the regulation of proopiomelanocortin (POMC) mRNA levels in the arcuate nucleus and pituitary gland of the female rat as studied by in situ hybridization. Brain Res Mol Brain Res 1992;15:27-32.

31. Gillard ER, Dang DQ, Stanley BG. Evidence that neuropeptide Y and dopamine in the perifornical hypothalamus interact antagonistically in the control of food intake. Brain Res 1993;628:128-136.

32. Baskin DG, Figlewicz Lattemann D, et al. Insulin and leptin: dual adiposity signals to the brain for the regulation of food intake and body weight. Brain Res 1999;848:114-123.

33. Meguid MM, Fetissov SO, Blaha V, et al. Dopamine and serotonin VMN release is related to feeding status in obese and lean Zucker rats. Neuroreport 2000; 11:2069-2072.

34. Balcioglu A, Wurtman RJ. Effects of phentermine on striatal dopamine and serotonin release in conscious rats: in vivo microdialysis study. Int J Obes Relat Metab Disord 1998;22:325-328.

35. Martel P, Fantino M. Mesolimbic dopaminergic system activity as a function of food reward: a microdialysis study. Pharmacol Biochem Behav 1996;53:221-226.

36. Pothos E, Creese I, Hoebel B. Restricted eating with weight loss selectively decreases extracellular dopamine in the nucleus accumbens and alters dopamine response to amphetamine, morphine, and food intake. J Neurosci 1995;15;6640-6650.

37. Berridge KC, Robinson TE. What is the role of dopamine in reward: hedonic impact, reward learning, or incentive salience? Brain Res Brain Res Rev 1998;28: 309-369.

38. Schwartz MW, Baskin DG, Kaiyala KJ, et al. Model for the regulation of energy balance and adiposity by the central nervous system. Am J Clin Nutr 1999;69:584-596.

39. Szczypka MS, Kwok K, Brot MD, et al. Dopamine production in the caudate putamen restores feeding in dopamine-deficient mice. Neuron 2001;30:819-828.

40. Bassareo V, Di Chiara G. Modulation of feeding-induced activation of mesolimbic dopamine transmission by appetitive stimuli and its relation to motivational state. Eur J Neurosci 1999;11:4389-4397.

41. Volkow ND, Wang G-J, Fowler JS, et al. "Nonhedonic" food motivation in humans involves dopamine in the dorsal striatum and methylphenidate amplifies this effect. Synapse 2002;44:175-180.

42. Spitzer RL, Yanovski S, Wadden T, et al. Binge eating disorder: its further validation in a multisite study. Int J Eat Disord 1993;13:137-153.

43. Goldfein JA, Walsh BT, LaChaussee JL, et al. Eating behavior in binge eating disorder. Int J Eat Disord 1993;14:427-431.

44. Yanovski SZ, Nelson JE, Dubbert BK, et al. Association of binge eating disorder and psychiatric comorbidity in obese subjects. Am J Psychiatry 1993;150:1472-1479.

45. Hsu LK, Sullivan SP, Benotti PN. Eating disturbances and outcome of gastric bypass surgery: a pilot study. Int J Eat Disord 1997;21:385-390.

46. Kalarchian MA, Wilson GT, Brolin RE, et al. Binge eating in bariatric surgery patients. Int J Eat Disord 1998;23:89-92.

47. Powers PS, Perez A, Boyd F, et al. Eating pathology before and after bariatric surgery: a prospective study. Int J Eat Disord 1999;25:293-300.

48. Saunders R. Binge eating in gastric bypass patients before surgery. Obes Surg 1999;9:72-76.

49. Dymek MP, le Grange D, Neven K, et al. Quality of life and psychosocial adjustment in patients after Roux-en-Y gastric bypass: a brief report. Obes Surg 2001; 11:32-39.

50. Kaye WH, Ballenger JC, Lydiard RB, et al. CSF monoamine levels in normal-weight bulimia: evidence for abnormal noradrenergic activity. Am J Psychiatry 1990;147:225-229.

51. Jimerson DC, Lesem MD, Kaye WH, et al. Low serotonin and dopamine metabolite concentrations in cerebrospinal fluid from bulimic patients with frequent binge episodes. Arch Gen Psychiatry 1992;49:132-138.

52. Noble EP, Noble RE, Ritchie T, et al. D2 dopamine receptor gene and obesity. Int J Eat Disord 1994;15:205-217.

53. Laruelle M, Gelernter J, Innis RB. D2 receptors binding potential is not affected by Taq1 polymorphism at the D2 receptor gene. Mol Psychiatry, 1998;3:261-265.

54. Noble EP, Blum K, Ritchie T, et al. Allelic association of the D2 dopamine receptor gene with receptor-binding characteristics in alcoholism. Arch Gen Psychiatry 1991;48:648-654.

55. Comings DE, Gade R, MacMurray JP, et al. Genetic variants of the human obesity (OB) gene: association with body mass index in young women, psychiatric symptoms, and interaction with the dopamine D2 receptor (DRD2) gene. Mol Psychiatry 1996;1:325-335.

56. Noble EP, Fitch RJ, Ritchie T, et al. The D2 dopamine receptor gene: obesity, smoking and mood. In: St. Jeor ST, ed. Obesity Assessment. Chapman and Hall; New York; 1997;pp522-533.

57. Scislowski PW, Tozzo E, Zhang Y, et al. Biochemical mechanisms responsible for the attenuation of diabetic and obese conditions in ob/ob mice treated with dopaminergic agonists. Int J Obes Relat Metab Disord 1999;23:425-431.

58. Allison DB, Casey DE. Antipsychotic-induced weight gain: a review of the literature. J Clin Psychiatry 2001;62Suppl7:22-31.

59. Wang G-J, Volkow ND, Logan J, et al. Brain dopamine and obesity. Lancet 2001;357:354-357.

60. Volkow ND, Wang G-J, Fowler JS, et al. Prediction of reinforcing responses to psychostimulants in humans by brain dopamine D2 receptor levels. Am J Psychiatry 1999;156:1440-1443.

61. Volkow ND, Wang G-J, Fowler JS, et al. Brain DA D2 receptors predict reinforcing effects of stimulants in humans: replication study. Synapse. 2002;46:79-82.

62. Patel KA, Schlundt DG. Impact of moods and social context on eating behavior. Appetite 2001;36:111-118.

63. Volkow ND, Fowler JS. Neuropsychiatric disorders: Investigation of schizophrenia and substance abuse. Sem Nucl Med 1992;12:254-267.

64. Wang G-J, Volkow ND, Fowler JS, et al. Enhanced Metabolism in Oral Regions of Somatosensory Cortex in Obese Individuals. NeuroReport 2002;13:1151-1155.

65. Urasaki E, Uematsu S, Gordon B, Lesser RP. Cortical tongue area studied by chronically implanted subdural electrodes–with special reference to parietal motor and frontal sensory responses. Brain 1994;117(Pt 1):117-132.

66. Drewnowski A. Intense sweeteners and energy density of foods: implications for weight control. Eur J Clin Nutr 1999;53:757-763.

67. Yeomans MR. Palatability and the micro-structure of feeding in humans: the appetizer effect. Appetite 1996;27:119-133.

68. Cooper SJ. Beta-carbolines characterized as benzodiazepine receptor agonists and inverse agonists produce bi-directional changes in palatable food consumption. Brain Res Bull 1986;17:627-37.

69. Yeomans MR, Gray RW. Effects of naltrexone on food intake and changes in subjective appetite during eating: evidence for opioid involvement in the appetizer effect. Physiol Behav 1997;62:15-21.

Adolescent Drug Addiction Treatment and Weight Gain

Candace C. Hodgkins, MA, LMHC
Kevin S. Cahill, BS
Anne E. Seraphine, PhD
Kimberly Frost-Pineda, MPH
Mark S. Gold, MD

SUMMARY. Neurotransmitter release in the nucleus accumbens use has been linked to self-administration and learning following drug use. This endogenous reward system is also activated following food intake or sex. Therefore, rebound hyperphagia following abstinence may be a mechanism to replenish the release of neurotransmitters in this reward system, leading to increased weight gain and a rise in Body Mass Index

Candace C. Hodgkins is Chief of Professional Services, Gateway Community Services, Inc., Jacksonville, Florida. Ms. Hodgkins is a doctoral candidate in the Department of Counselor Education at the University of Florida, Gainesville, FL.

Kevin S. Cahill is a MD/PhD student at the University of Florida, Gainesville, FL.

Anne E. Seraphine is Assistant Professor, Department of Educational Psychology, University of Florida College of Education, Gainesville, FL.

Kimberly Frost-Pineda is Coordinator, Research Programs/Services, Division of Addiction Medicine, University of Florida College of Medicine.

Mark S. Gold is Distinguished Professor, Departments of Psychiatry, Neuroscience, Community Health & Family Medicine, and Chief of Addiction Medicine, University of Florida College of Medicine, Gainesville, FL.

Address correspondence to: Candace C. Hodgkins, Gateway Community Services, Inc., 555 Stockton Street, Jacksonville, FL 32224.

[Haworth co-indexing entry note]: "Adolescent Drug Addiction Treatment and Weight Gain." Hodgkins, Candace C. et al. Co-published simultaneously in *Journal of Addictive Diseases* (The Haworth Medical Press, an imprint of The Haworth Press, Inc.) Vol. 23, No. 3, 2004, pp. 55-65; and: *Eating Disorders, Overeating, and Pathological Attachment to Food: Independent or Addictive Disorders?* (ed: Mark S. Gold) The Haworth Medical Press, an imprint of The Haworth Press, Inc., 2004, pp. 55-65. Single or multiple copies of this article are available for a fee from The Haworth Document Delivery Service [1-800-HAWORTH, 9:00 a.m. - 5:00 p.m. (EST). E-mail address: docdelivery@haworthpress.com].

http://www.haworthpress.com/web/JAD
© 2004 by The Haworth Press, Inc. All rights reserved.
Digital Object Identifer: 10.1300/J069v23n03_05

during recovery from substance abuse. In this report, we examined the relationship between supervised drug abstinence and increased weight gain among adolescents at a residential substance abuse treatment center. Mean weight change over time was followed by repeated analysis of weight and body mass index. Significant weight gain and body mass index increase was observed during supervised and confirmed abstinence from drug use. Furthermore, significant interactions between tobacco use and primary substance use disorder with weight gain was demonstrated by multivariate analysis of variance. *[Article copies available for a fee from The Haworth Document Delivery Service: 1-800-HAWORTH. E-mail address: <docdelivery@haworthpress.com> Website: <http://www.HaworthPress. com> © 2004 by The Haworth Press, Inc. All rights reserved.]*

KEYWORDS. Adolescents, addiction, weight, BMI, drugs

INTRODUCTION

Substance Abuse and Adolescents

The use of tobacco, alcohol, and illicit drugs by adolescents has risen for most of the past two decades, with a plateau and then significant declines since 1999.[1] However, the percentage of adolescents using alcohol and drugs in the U.S. remains shockingly high. According to the 1996 annual Monitoring the Future (MTF) Study,[2] about one-third of high school seniors reported being drunk in the past month, while one-fifth of 10th and 12th graders used marijuana in that same time period. MTF data from 2002 shows that seniors who reported using alcohol on a daily basis increased from 2.9 percent in 2000 to 3.5 percent in 2002, and past year marijuana use by seniors was at 36.2 percent in 2002.[3]

In addition to high rates of use, adolescents are using substances of abuse at younger and younger ages,[3] often initiating use between the ages of 10 to13 with cigarettes, alcohol and then moving to experimentation with marijuana and club drugs.[4] The 2002 MFT report cited 8.3% of 8th graders, 17.8% of 10th graders, and 21.5% of 12th graders as current users of marijuana, which, along with tobacco and alcohol, is often called a "gateway drug" to other illicit drug use.[5,6] While marijuana is the most widely used illicit drug, many adolescents report the use of poly-substances. In recent years, the club drug "ecstasy" (MDMA) increased dramatically. Johnston et al.[1] reported that use of ecstasy by eighth graders rose from 1.7% in 1999 to 3.5% in 2001, while use among 10th and 12th graders increased to almost 10%, making it a drug that is more frequently used than cocaine by adolescents.

Overweight and Obese Adolescents

The prevalence of adult and adolescent obesity has increased at alarming rates in the past three decades. In fact, adolescent obesity has been described by the Centers for Disease Control and Prevention (CDC) as an epidemic.[7] This striking increase has been linked to the dramatic rise in Type II Diabetes among young persons. Today, one out of every five youths in the U.S. is overweight [7] and one in four is at risk of becoming overweight.[8] Among adults, half are overweight and almost one-quarter suffers from obesity. This translates to approximately 97 million overweight adults and about 40 million obese adults.[9] The remarkable increase in obesity among adolescents in the U.S. has resulted in recommendations for more exercise, food restriction, and even bariatric surgery.[10] Complications of childhood obesity include psychosocial, psychological, neurological, cardiovascular, endocrine, musculoskeletal, renal, gastrointestinal, and pulmonary problems.[11]

Overweight is defined as an increase in weight relative to some standard. Obesity is defined as an excessively high amount of body fat or adipose tissue in relation to lean body mass. Body fat distribution can be estimated by a variety of techniques. The three most common techniques for evaluating body weight are life insurance tables, relative weight (actual weight/desirable weight $\times$ 100), and Body Mass Index (BMI). The standard definition of overweight adults is having a BMI (calculated by weight in kilograms/height in meters squared) between the 85th and 95th percentile, with severe obesity in adults being any BMI greater than the 95th percentile. Calculating BMI is simple and it correlates well with clinical measures, which is why it is commonly used in epidemiological studies. Although there are some exceptions, a BMI above 25 (overweight) and above 30 (obese), is a useful guide to estimate the degree of excess fat and health risk.[12]

For children and adolescents, the CDC recommend using specific charts of calculated BMI values for selected heights and weight for ages 2 to 20 years.[13] This is due to the change in body fatness as the child ages and develops. CDC defines "at-risk for becoming overweight" as having a BMI between the 85th percentile and the 95th percentile for a person's age and gender. Any BMI over the 95th percentile is considered overweight trending toward obesity.

Substance Abuse and Eating Disorders

A recent report from SAMHSA[14] suggests there is a strong correlation among youth between substance abuse and several behavioral and emotional problems. However, little current research focuses on substance use and weight gain, obesity, or eating disorders. In one recent study by Ross and Ivis,[15] binge eaters were more likely to use all types of substances and a high correlation was found for cannabis use. Adolescent eating disorders and substance abuse are both major public health issues in the U.S. The cost to society for health care related to these problems is extraordinary. Adolescents who are obese and those that are substance dependent often continue to have these problems as adults. Weight in adolescence is a predictor of adult weight[16] and later adverse health events, as is substance abuse a predictor of future substance abuse and dependence.

We have previously reported that adolescents in a supervised treatment setting gained significant weight while abstinent from alcohol and illicit drugs. Thus it appears important that further research address the particular variables associated with the phenomena, with particular attention to improved treatment program development.

Tobacco Use and Weight Gain

It has been demonstrated that smokers have a propensity to gain weight when they quit smoking, although on average there is only a 6-8 pound gain for each individual when they quit.[17] Weight gain in the adult population has been found to be statistically significant over a 10 year period for those individuals who quit smoking versus those individuals who had never smoked,[18] therefore suggesting that the increase in overweight individuals in the Untied States may be slightly associated with the increase of smoking cessation during that period of time. Research suggests that adult women have a more difficult time of quitting smoking and are more prone to relapse due to weight concerns.[19] It also appears that concern about weight gain is correlated with fewer quit attempts and minimal intentions to quit.[20]

Given the various relationships between appetite, taste, drugs of abuse, brain reward pathways and eating disorders, as well as the widespread occurrence of adolescent obesity, many factors must be considered by treatment providers to enhance and refine current modalities regarding adolescent substance abuse treatment. The purpose of this study was to further clarify the relationship of weight gain to abstinence from drug use in adolescents. This was accomplished through the analysis of 75 adolescent patients admitted to a residential substance abuse treatment facility between 1999 and 2002. Data obtained from these patients were used to test the following hypotheses:

1. There is significant weight increase during supervised treatment and abstinence from alcohol, illicit drugs, and tobacco.
2. There is an interaction effect between weight increase and smoking.
3. There is an interaction effect between BMI increase and smoking.
4. There is an interaction effect between weight increase and primary drug of choice.
5. There is an interaction effect between BMI increase and primary drug of choice.

METHODS

Source of Data and Sample

This study was conducted at an adolescent residential substance abuse treatment center in a southeastern city in the United States. The facility is a 24-bed substance abuse treatment center for males and females, ages 13 through 17. This population of adolescents is referred to the treatment program by three different means: self-referral, civil commitment by parents, or adjudicated by the court system. The adolescent participants in this program are supervised on the campus twenty-four hours a day, seven days a week with the average length of stay amounting to 168 days. The center is a non-secure facility. All participants are required to abstain from all alcohol, illicit drug use and tobacco during time of treatment. Drug screens are obtained when participants leave campus for any reason and participants are also randomly tested during their stay at the facility. All information for this study was obtained from existing data sets held in reserve for outcome measures by the organization. Each participant in treatment signs a consent form giving the organization permission to use data from the charts for research purposes, by qualified individuals, with the understanding that all identifying information will be kept confidential. This research project was reviewed and approved by the University of Florida Institutional Review Board.

A total of 215 male (n = 148) and female (n = 67) patients were involved in treatment for varying lengths of time from the beginning of August 1999 until the end of July 2002. The mean age for the sample was 15.8 years. The majority of the patients were male (n = 109; 70.3%), whereas almost thirty percent were female (n = 46; 29.7%). The group consisted of 80.1% non-Hispanic white and 17.9% African American patients, with the remaining 1.9% of patients from other ethnicities. There was a higher percentage of smokers, 82.4%, than non-smokers, 17.6%. Patients diagnosed according to DSM-IV criteria for cannabis abuse equaled 19.2%, cannabis dependence equaled 57.7%, and polysubstance abuse equaled 23.2%. After excluding patients in treatment for fewer than thirty days and patients with incomplete data sets, 75 patients were randomly chosen for inclusion in this analysis.

Analysis

For this two between subjects factor (i.e., smoking and SUD) and one within subjects factor (time in treatment: admit date, 60 days, 90 days, and discharge) design, the most suitable statistical procedure was a multivariate analysis of variance. Although there were a total of eight different primary SUD diagnoses reported in this patient population, only those diagnoses that equaled more than 10 in a cell were analyzed. The SUD's meeting that criterion were Cannabis Abuse, Cannabis Dependence, and Poly-Substance Dependence. For this study, SPSS was used for the statistical analysis. All statistical tests were conducted at $\alpha = .05$.

RESULTS

Two separate MANOVAs were conducted, one for each of the two outcome measures: weight and BMI. The results of the MANOVAs are reported in Tables 1 and 2 for weight and BMI, respectively. For each outcome variable, time in treatment and the interaction between smoking and time in treatment were statistically significant. These two effects were also practically significant, given that the eta squared values showed both effects to be large according to Cohen's[21] criterion.

The descriptive statistics for weight and BMI are reported in Table 3. There was a substantial weight gain and BMI increase from admittance to 60 days. Participants gained an average of about 11 pounds and in-

TABLE 1. MANOVA for Weight

Effect	Pillai's Trace	F	df	p	Eta Squared
Time	.515	23.69	3,67	.00	.515
Time*Smoke	.127	3.26	3,67	.03	.127
Time*Drug	.131	1.58	6,136	.16	.065
Time*Smoke*Drug	.065	.76	6,136	.61	.032

TABLE 2. MANOVA for BMI

Effect	Pillai's Trace	F	df	p	Eta Squared
Time	.469	19.72	3,67	.00	.469
Time*Smoke	.123	3.15	3,67	.03	.123
Time*Drug	.153	1.87	6,136	.09	.076
Time*Smoke*Drug	.044	.51	6,136	.80	.022

creased their BMI by 1.58 during this time. Mean weight gain was less from 60 days to discharge. In addition to weight and BMI, Table 3 indicates the percentage of the patients who are at-risk for being overweight and those who are overweight. The CDC defines at-risk for becoming overweight as having a BMI between the 85th percentile and the 95th percentile for a person's age and gender. Consequently, by definition, 10% of the population would be expected to be at-risk for becoming overweight. The percent of patients at-risk for becoming overweight increased after admittance to the program, going from 7.1% at admittance and increasing to 14.7%, a percentage that is above the expected 10% for a gender and age matched population. Similarly, CDC defines being overweight as having a BMI above the 95th percentile for a person's age and gender. Again, this definition leads to an expectation that 5% of the population is overweight. Upon admittance, the sample was slightly higher (5.8%) than expected for the population (5%). At 60 days, the percent overweight was almost double the population expectation. By the time of discharge, the percent overweight was 2.7 times the expected (13.5/5 = 2.7). Table 3 shows a clear trend toward weight gain for participants in the program, especially during the first 60 days of treatment.

Descriptive statistics for effect of smoking on weight gain are reported in Table 4. The means for weight and BMI gain show substantial gains only from admission to 60 days. The interaction is due to the

TABLE 3. Descriptive Statistics for Weight and BMI Over Time

	Admit	60-Day	90-Day	Discharge
Weight – Mean	147.91	160.27	165.57	160.19
– (SD)	(31.27)	(32.22)	(31.18)	(30.90)
BMI – Mean	23.26	24.90	25.03	25.00
– (SD)	(4.84)	(4.65)	(4.23)	(4.63)
% At-Risk for Overweight*	7.1	12.2	14.7	13.5
% Overweight*	5.8	9.6	10.3	13.5

*At-risk for being overweight is defined by the CDC as being between the 85% and 95% for the appropriate age and gender; Overweight is defined as being above the 95 percentile for the appropriate age and gender.

TABLE 4. Means for Weight and BMI by Smoking

	Admit	60-Day	90-Day	Discharge
Weight				
Smoking	147.63	161.99	167.83	160.16
Non-Smoking	145.06	153.74	152.56	156.91
BMI				
Smoking	23.37	25.16	25.26	25.18
Non-Smoking	22.23	23.90	23.58	23.80

larger weight and BMI gain for adolescents who smoked prior to treatment.

DISCUSSION

This study demonstrates that there is significant weight and BMI increase while adolescents are residing in a supervised substance abuse treatment setting. It is evident that both weight gain and BMI over time are influenced by weather or not the individual smokes prior to treatment. The rate of weight and BMI gain from 0-60 days was the highest for smokers. No interaction effect for primary diagnosis was shown. These data suggest that adolescents who smoke are at greater risk of weight gain during supervised abstinence from drugs, including tobacco, and alcohol, increasing their propensity to become at risk of being overweight.

Regardless of the initial external decisions that prompted drug use, once in the body the drug promotes continued drug seeking behavior. The impact of drugs, tobacco, and alcohol on the brain is modulated by reinforcement and neuroadaptation that contribute to the process of addiction. The ventral tegmental area and the basal forebrain contain the general reward circuitry and the use of drugs can change the neural processes around these connections. These two areas are connected by the mesolimbic dopamine system that is critical to the self-administration of psychomotor stimulants[22] with motivational behavior acting as a crucial function.[23] Food, tobacco, and illicit drugs are all reported to be addictive or stimulating to the brain reward system.[24] Food ingestion, as well as smoking and other drug self-administration, is linked to the neurotransmitter dopamine and is the subject of current studies.[25-27]

It has been suggested that individuals who are prone to drug or food addiction may have a deficiency of dopamine. Wang et al.[27] tested the hypothesis that obese individuals have abnormalities in brain dopamine activity. They determined that striatal dopamine receptor (DRD2) availability was significantly lower in obese individuals than in the control group. The BMI correlated negatively with the measures of D2 receptors, suggesting that individuals with the largest BMI had the lowest D2 values. Thanos et al.[28] studied ethanol preferring rats over-expressing the DRD2. Their results suggest that an increase in DRD2 results in reductions in alcohol preference and alcohol intake. These two molecular studies underscore the concept that the under-expression of dopamine receptors in the brain may lead to both food and drug addiction. These findings support the necessity of further examining the issue of weight gain during supervised drug abstinence and the influence of other factors such as tobacco status.

Adolescence is a time of numerous developmental changes from various influences. Adolescence is also a time of self-consciousness about body image and perceived looks, influenced by the power of being accepted or rejected by peers.[29] In this study, 36.1% of adolescents entered treatment either underweight or at normal weight, while only 21.9% remained in this category at discharge. It is possible to speculate that tobacco and illicit drugs may be partially sought as a weight control measure. Therefore, an inordinate amount of weight gain during treatment may lead to depression and may be viewed as a significant relapse issue that must be addressed. There are also numerous physical complications of excessive weight gain, such as heart disease, breathing, and joint problems, and the dramatic increase in Type II diabetes (previously called "adult onset diabetes"), which until recently was almost non-existent in children and adolescents.[11]

This study has widespread implications for the field of addiction medicine when determining treatment protocols and assessing adolescents during treatment. Treatment providers pay close attention to dealing with alcohol, tobacco, and illicit drug use in the treatment settings, but the effects of abstinence on weight gain are not addressed. Most programs do not spend significant time on nutritional counseling, exercise, and education concerning the substitution of food for drugs of choice. Further research is needed to examine effective treatment protocols in these areas. Larger data sets with both smokers and non-smokers, females, ethnic populations, and the effects of co-occurring disorders treated with medication may be explored to address the relationship of appetite, drug withdrawal, and coping in an adolescent population.

REFERENCES

1. Johnston LD, O'Malley PM, Bachman JG. The Monitoring the future national results on adolescent drug use, 1975-2000. 2001. Bethesda, Maryland: U.S. Department of Health and Human Services, National Institutes of Health; 2000.

2. Johnston LD, O'Malley PM, Bachman JG. The Monitoring the future national results on adolescent drug use: Overview of key findings. 1995. Bethesda, Maryland: U.S. Department of Health and Human Services, National Institutes of Health; 1996.

3. American Academy of Pediatrics, Committee on Substance Abuse. Alcohol use and abuse: A pediatric concern. Pediatrics 2001;108:185-189.

4. Johnson PB, Boles SM, Kleber HD. The relationship between adolescent smoking and drinking and likelihood estimates of illicit drug use. J Addictiv Dis. 2000; 19:75-81.

5.. Lai S, Lai H, Page JB, et al. The association between cigarette smoking and drug abuse in the United States. J Addictiv Dis. 2000; 19:11-24.

6. Weinberg NZ, Rahdert E, Colliver JD. Adolescent substance abuse: A review of the past 10 years. J Am Acad Child Adolesc Psychiatry. 1998;37:252-261.

7. Dietz W. Childhood obesity. In: Shils M, Olsen J, Shike M, et al., editors. Modern Nutrition in Health and Disease. Ninth edition. Baltimore: Williams and Wilkins; 1999. pp. 1071-1080.

8. CDC. Youth risk behavioral surveillance. Atlanta: Centers for Disease Control; 2000.

9. Cunningham E, Marcason W. Obesity update. J Am Diet Assoc. 2001;101:80.

10. Yanovski JA. Intensive therapies for pediatric obesity. Ped Clin Nor Amer. 2001;48:1041-1053.

11. Ebbeling CB, Pawlak DB, Ludwig DS. Childhood obesity: Public-health crisis, common sense cure. Lancet. 2002; 360:473-482.

12. Bray GA, Bouchard C, James WP, editors. Handbook of Obesity. New York: Marcel Dekker; 1997.

13. CDC. (2000). Body mass index-for-age: BMI is used differently with children than it is with adults. Retrieved 9-2, 2002, from *http://www.cdc.gov/nccdphp/dnpa/ bmi/bmi-for-age.htm*

14. SAMHSA. SAMHSA study links behavior problems, alcohol use. Brown Univ Dig Addict Theory Appl. 2000;19: 5-6.

15. Ross HE, Ivis F. Binge eating and substance use among male and female adolescents. Inter J Eat Dis. 1999;26:245-260.

16. Whitaker RC, Wright JA, Pepe MS. Predicting obesity in young adulthood from childhood and parental weight. NEJW. 1997;337:869-873.

17. Fact Sheet No.11. (2001). What happens when you stop smoking. Available: *http://www.ash.org.uk/html/factsheets/html/fact11/html*; accessed 1/16/03.

18. Flegal KM, Troiano RP, Pamuk ER, et al. The influence of smoking cessation on the prevalence of overweight in the United States. NEJM. 1995; 333: 1165-1170.

19. Pomerleau CS, Pomerleau OF, Namenek RJ, Mehringer BA. Short-term weight gain in abstaining women smokers. J Subst Abuse Treat. 2000; 18:339-342.

20. Weekley CK, Klesges RC, Relyea G. Smoking as a weight control strategy and its relationship to smoking status. Addict Behav. 1992; 17:259-271.

21. Cohen J. Statistical Power Analysis for the Behavioral Sciences (2nd ed.). Mahwak, New Jersey: Laurence Erlbaum Associates, 1988.

22. Roberts AJ, Koob GF. The neurobiology of addiction: An overview. Alcohol Health & Res World 1997;21: 101-106.

23. Tenth Special Report to the United States Congress on Alcohol and Health. Alcohol, the brain, and behavior: Mechanisms of addiction. Alcohol Research & Health 2000;24:12-15.

24. Gold MS, Johnson C, Stennie K. Eating disorders. In Substance Abuse: A Comprehensive Textbook. Ninth edition, Lowenstein JH, Ruiz P, Millman RB, Langrod JD (eds.). Baltimore: Williams and Wilkins. 1997. pp. 319-330.

25. Linseman MA, Harding S. Alcohol consumption following bidirectional shifts in body weight in rats. Psychopharmacology 1989; 97:103-107.

26. NIDA. 2001. Dopamine receptors implicated in obesity. Available *http:// www.nida.nih.gov*; Accessed 7-19-01.

27. Wang GJ, Volkow ND, Logan J, et al. Brain dopamine and obesity. Lancet. 2001; 357:354-357.

28. Thanos PK, Volkow ND, Freimuth P, et al. Overexpression of dopamine D2 receptors reduces alcohol self-administration. J Neurochem. 2001; 78:1094-1103.

29. Nowinski J. Substance Abuse in Adolescents and Young Adults. New York: W.W. Norton and Company, 1990.

Examining Problem Drinking and Eating Disorders from a Gendered Perspective

Connie R. Matthews, PhD

SUMMARY. The two studies presented here examined the relationship between problem drinking and eating disorders in college students. Although there was little evidence of a concurrent relationship between the two, there were differences related to gender. In addition, there were differences between women who were and were not sorority members with respect to problem drinking, but not eating disorders. The value of addressing these problems from a gendered perspective is discussed. *[Article copies available for a fee from The Haworth Document Delivery Service: 1-800-HAWORTH. E-mail address: <docdelivery@haworthpress.com> Website: <http://www.HaworthPress.com> © 2004 by The Haworth Press, Inc. All rights reserved.]*

KEYWORDS. Alcohol, eating, disorder, gender, college

Both eating disorders and problem drinking among college students have received much attention in recent years. It is difficult to precisely

Connie R. Matthews, Department of Counselor Education, Counseling Psychology and Rehabilitation Services, 333 CEDAR Building, The Pennsylvania State University, University Park, PA 16802 (E-mail: cxm206@psu.edu).

[Haworth co-indexing entry note]: "Examining Problem Drinking and Eating Disorders from a Gendered Perspective." Matthews, Connie R. Co-published simultaneously in *Journal of Addictive Diseases* (The Haworth Medical Press, an imprint of The Haworth Press, Inc.) Vol. 23, No. 3, 2004, pp. 67-80; and: *Eating Disorders, Overeating, and Pathological Attachment to Food: Independent or Addictive Disorders?* (ed: Mark S. Gold) The Haworth Medical Press, an imprint of The Haworth Press, Inc., 2004, pp. 67-80. Single or multiple copies of this article are available for a fee from The Haworth Document Delivery Service [1-800-HAWORTH, 9:00 a.m. - 5:00 p.m. (EST). E-mail address: docdelivery@haworthpress.com].

http://www.haworthpress.com/web/JAD
© 2004 by The Haworth Press, Inc. All rights reserved.
Digital Object Identifer: 10.1300/J069v23n03_06

determine the prevalence of either problem due to differences in measurement between studies, but it is possible to discern some patterns. For instance, the literature has consistently reported patterns of heavier, more frequent, more problematic use by men than by women.[1-4] Conversely, estimates suggest that about 90% of individuals with eating disorders are women.[5] Still, there are some methodological concerns.

One difficulty lies with reports of consumption patterns. Such reports rarely take into account differences in body weight between men and women.[1,6] With generally lower body weight, women may actually experience alcohol similarly to men at lower levels of consumption. Ratliff and Burkhart[7] found support for this when initial differences in alcohol intake between college men and women disappeared when they controlled for weight. Conversely, others[8,9] did find significant gender differences in rates of binge drinking even when adjustments were made.

Sociocultural factors also operate differently for women than they do for men. While social proscriptions operate against excessive drinking in women, they are more permissive, if not encouraging, for men especially in college.[2,6,10,11] Burns and Sloane[6] point out that these differences also "subtly shift our focus to behavior that is more social and more boisterous." Perhaps it is not that college men experience more problems due to drinking, but that they experience different problems and those problems more frequently catch our attention.

Perkins[11] found that college men more frequently experienced difficulties that were public and disruptive, however, women were as or more likely to experience consequences that were less public, involving harm to self rather than others. Others[10,12] have also found college men more likely than college women to experience consequences that could be considered disruptive. Moos et al.[13] found heavy drinking college women showed greater negative affect than their abstaining peers on every measure, while heavy drinking college males differed from abstaining males on only a few of those measures. Similarly, Reiskin and Wechsler[14] found that women using a campus mental health center showed higher levels of alcohol use than women in the general campus population, while men using the mental health center showed generally lower patterns of use than men in the larger group. Robbins[15] examined sex differences in the consequences of drug and alcohol use and found that, controlling for level of use, females showed greater psychological consequences, while males showed more social and behavioral problems.

Horowitz and White[16] suggested that males and females exhibit different styles of pathology. They found that males showed greater levels of delinquent behaviors and alcohol and drug problems and females showed greater levels of psychological distress. Oliver et al.[17] also found that males experienced "acting out or rule-violating types of maladjustment," while females experienced "internalizing behaviors accompanied by high levels of subjective distress."

A number of researchers have argued a link between eating disorders and chemical dependency, especially in women, with food as the substance of choice.[18-21] They suggest parallels between eating disorders and chemical dependency that include symptomatology, etiology, assessment, intervention, and approaches to treatment, as well as physiological similarities in reactions to the presence or deprivation of both food and drugs.

Like problem drinking, eating disorders are a serious concern on college campuses.[22] A number of studies[23-25] have looked at implications of this. They found college women with eating disorders, especially bulimia, to be more depressed than college women without eating disorders. Wechsler et al.[26] found problems with weight control to be related to a variety of affective symptoms in both college males and females, although they reported almost five times the percentage of females as males expressing such concerns. These studies seem to indicate a pattern with eating disorders similar to what Perkins[11] reported with substance abuse–women with symptomatic or disordered behavior turning their turmoil inward in a manner that increases the problems they experience personally but is not socially disruptive.

A limited number of investigations have examined the relationship between eating disorders and alcoholism in college women. Lundholm[27] found significant differences between those who scored high and those who scored low on the Alcohol Abuse Scale of the Millon Clinical Multiaxial Inventory (MCMI) on five subscales of the Eating Disorders Inventory (EDI), including Interoceptive Awareness, Ineffectiveness, Maturity Fears, Interpersonal Distrust, and Bulimia. Kashubeck and Mintz[28] found significant but weak relationships between problematic drinking and the Bulimia and Interoceptive Awareness subscales of the EDI in a sample of college women. Since problem drinking and eating disorders pose serious concerns on college campuses, it is important to continue investigation in this area and to begin examining both problems from a perspective that takes gender into account.

The first part of this study addressed the prevalence of both eating disorders and problem drinking in a general undergraduate population.

The first research question asked whether there would be significant differences between men and women in rates of problem drinking and rates of eating disorder symptomatology. Although the existing literature is somewhat consistent in suggesting that problem drinking is greater among college men and eating disorders are more frequent among college women, there have not been studies that examined both issues concurrently among both males and females. This study did that. Based on the previous literature, it was predicted that a higher percentage of men would score positively for problem drinking and a higher percentage of women would score positively for eating disorders.

The second part of the study focused on women. It examined more closely whether there was a relationship between problem drinking and eating disorders in college women. The second research question asked whether there would be a significant positive relationship between those who scored positively on a screening instrument for problem drinking and those who scored positively on a screening instrument for eating disorders. It was predicted that there would be. The third research question asked whether there would be a significant positive relationship between positive scores on a screening instrument for problem drinking and specific subscales of the Eating Disorders Inventory-2. Based on the Lundholm[27] and Kashubeck and Mintz[28] studies, it was predicted that problem drinkers would score higher on the Bulimia, Interoceptive Awareness, Ineffectiveness, Maturity Fears, and Interpersonal Distrust subscales. It was also predicted that they would score higher on the Impulse Regulation subscale since this was a new subscale added to the EDI-2 specifically to tap this dimension.

METHODS

Participants

Participants were 289 traditionally aged (18-25)-college students at a large mid-Atlantic university. They were mostly Caucasian (93%), which was reflective of the university, with very small percentages of African American, Asian/Pacific Islander, Hispanic/Latino, Non-U.S. National, or other. The entire sample was 78% female (N = 225) and 22% male (N = 64), however, this was broken down for the comparison of males and females in the first research question (see Procedures). The mean age was 20.32. Freshmen were underrepresented, however, sophomores, juniors, and seniors were somewhat proportionately represented.

Instruments

Alcohol Use Disorders Identification Test (AUDIT). The full AUDIT[29,30] consists of two parts, a ten-item, self-report, pencil and paper screening instrument and a screening interview. The written portion was used for this study. The ten items include two quantity-frequency questions, one item related to binge drinking, two CAGE questions, and five questions based on DSM III criteria. There are five multiple-choice type responses for each item, with scores on each item ranging from zero to four, with higher scores reflecting more problematic behavior. The highest possible score for the instrument is 40. Flemming et al.[31] found that a cut-off score of >13 had better predictive values for college students than the 8 or 10 originally recommended by the developers,[29] so that was used for this study. In a clinical setting a positive score would be reflective of problematic drinking that would suggest the need for a more extensive diagnostic procedure.

The AUDIT was developed to measure hazardous and harmful drinking, not the more extreme alcohol dependence, which is important when considering use with college students. Using a cut-off score of >13 with college students, Flemming et al.[31] reported sensitivity for the AUDIT to be .70, specificity .78, positive predictive value .57, negative predictive value .86, and a likelihood ratio of 3.18.

Eating Disorders Inventory-2 (EDI-2). The EDI-2,[32] is a multifaceted self-report questionnaire designed to assess the psychological and behavioral traits often found in people with anorexia nervosa and bulimia. The EDI-2 retains the original 64 items and eight subscales from the original EDI and has an additional 27 items that factor onto three new provisional subscales. The original subscales are Drive for Thinness (DT), Bulimia (B), Body Dissatisfaction (BD), Ineffectiveness (I), Perfectionism (P), Interpersonal Distrust (ID), Interoceptive Awareness (IA), and Maturity Fears (MF). The new provisional subscales are Asceticism (A), Impulse Regulation (IR), and Social Insecurity (SI).

Items contain statements about behaviors or attitudes. The individual responds on a six-point Likert scale according to the degree to which the statement applies to her or him. Response choices are always, usually, often, sometimes, rarely, and never. For each item, three responses are asymptomatic and are not scored. Scores of 3, 2, or 1 are given for the three responses indicating eating disorder symptomatology, with more symptomatic responses receiving higher points. Some items are scored in the positive direction and some are scored in the negative direction.

Each item is scored on only one subscale. Subscale scores are totaled and plotted on a Profile Sheet. No overall score is given. The individual's profile is compared to the profile for the eating disorder norm group and the college student comparison norm group. Six counseling psychology doctoral students trained in the use and scoring of the EDI-2 served as raters to classify profiles as symptomatic of an eating disorder or non-symptomatic. There was consensus on all profiles.

According to the EDI-2 Manual,[32] the internal consistency reliability coefficients for all of the original eight subscales are .80 or above for eating disorder samples and range from .65 (MF) to .93 (BD) for nonpatient comparison groups. Most were above .80. Internal consistency for the three provisional scales ranged from .70 to .80 for the eating disorder group and from .44 to .80 for the nonpatient comparison group.

Background Questionnaire. This was a nine item questionnaire developed by the author to gather descriptive information about the sample.

Procedures

Participation was voluntary and anonymous. Due to the fact that problem drinking and eating disorders are sensitive topics, the description of the study was kept general. Students were told that the study was examining attitudes and behaviors of college students. Upon completion of the instruments, participants were given debriefing sheets that described the study more specifically and provided information about resources available on campus for those who might be concerned about their own behavior.

The instruments were administered to male and female undergraduates in introductory educational psychology and introductory counselor education courses. As introductory courses, all of the classes tended to attract students from a variety of majors. A small number of participants completed the instruments in an out of class administration in response to flyers posted in residence halls and classroom buildings. A total of 218 students (154 females; 64 males) completed the instruments through this approach. This sample was used for the first research question, which compared male and female prevalence rates for each problem.

The instruments were administered to an additional 71 women in sorority meetings. This approach was used to increase the number of women participants available for the multivariate analysis for the third research question and to allow comparison between women who are and are not members of a sorority. Previous research has found greater levels and frequencies of problem drinking and eating disorders among women in sororities than in the general student population.[33,34]

RESULTS

Preliminary analysis found that all participants could be classified according to problem status. The first part of the study looked at both men and women. The sample included 154 women and 64 men who completed the instruments in class or during an out of class administration. The first research question asked whether there were significant differences between men and women in rates of problem drinking and rates of eating disorder symptomatology. A 2 × 2 chi square analysis looking at problem drinking status by gender was significant (X^2 = 5.027; df = 1; p = .025). Males were more likely to report problem drinking. Seventeen and two-tenth percent (17.2%) of the males scored positively on the AUDIT, compared to 7.1% of the women. A 2 × 2 chi square analysis looking at eating disorder status by gender was also significant (X^2 = 7.392; df = 1; p = .007). Females were more likely to report eating disorder symptomatology. Twenty-one and four-tenth percent (21.4%) of the women scored positively on the EDI-2, compared to 6.3% of the males.

The second part of the study addressed only women. It included the 154 described above and an additional 71 women who completed the instruments in sorority meetings. The second research question asked whether there was a significant relationship between problem drinking and eating disorders in college women. A 2 × 2 chi square analysis examined problem drinking status against eating disorder status. The results showed no significant relationship (X^2 = .471; df = 1; p = .492). Eight and nine-tenth percent (8.9%) of the women scored positively for problem drinking alone, 17.8% scored positively for eating disorder symptomatology alone, and 3.1% scored positively for both.

The third research question asked whether there was a significant relationship between problem drinking and specific subscales of the EDI-2. A 2 × 11 multivariate analysis of variance (MANOVA) was used to examine the independent variable of problem drinking status (problem versus non-problem drinking) against scores on each of the eleven subscales of the EDI-2, which served as the dependent variables. This analysis was conducted on 219 participants. Six participants did not complete several items on the three provisional subscales and were not included in the analysis. Since these subscales are considered provisional and skipped items did not effect any other subscales or other instruments, a decision was made not to eliminate these participants completely from the study. Due to the provisional nature of the subscales, raters had been instructed to give more weight to the original subscales in making categorical determinations, so skipped items primarily affected subscale scores. Furthermore, all skipped items were on the back of a page, more likely overlooked by participants than systematically avoided.

The overall MANOVA was significant at the .05 level [Wilks' Lambda = 0.91, F (11, 207) = 1.86, p = .05]. The univariate tests on each of the subscales revealed that only the Impulse Regulation (IR) subscale was significant (F = 11.38, df = 1, p = .0009).

Because the literature has suggested that women who are in sororities are more likely than women in the general campus population to experience both problem drinking and eating disorders, additional analysis was done to compare these two groups. In response to a question on the Background Questionnaire, 46.7% of the women indicated that they were currently members of a sorority and 52.9% indicated that they were not currently members of a sorority. Two 2 × 2 chi square analyses examined sorority status (in a sorority vs. not in a sorority) against problem drinking status and against eating disorder symptomatology status. The relationship between sorority status and eating disorder symptomatology status was not significant at the .05 level (chi square value = 0.04, df = 1, p = .85). Among sorority members, 11.16% scored positively on the EDI-2. Among non-sorority members, 9.38% scored positively on the EDI-2. There was a significant relationship between sorority status and problem drinking status, with a greater percentage of sorority members scoring positively on the AUDIT (chi square value = 6.81, df = 1, p = .009). Higher percentage of sorority members (8.48%) scored positively on the AUDIT compared to 3.57% of non-sorority members.

DISCUSSION

The first part of the study compared male and female undergraduates with respect to prevalence rates of problem drinking and eating disorder symptomatology as measured by the AUDIT and the EDI-2. While the existing literature has suggested that males more frequently experience problem drinking and females more frequently experience eating disor-

ders, there have not been studies that have examined both problems together in both males and females. The present study did this and, not
surprisingly, found higher prevalence of problem drinking among males
and higher prevalence of eating disorder symptomatology among females. What is interesting in looking at both issues concurrently in both
males and females is that the percentage of participants involved in specific behaviors was almost reversed by gender. In other words, there
seemed to be similar percentages of males and females screening positively for problem behavior, however, the problem they experienced
seemed somewhat gender specific.

The second part of the study looked more closely at women undergraduates in particular. The second research question asked whether
there would be a significant positive relationship between scoring positively for problem drinking and scoring positively for eating disorder
symptomatology. That relationship was not significant. Although 8.9%
of the women participants scored positively for problem drinking alone
and 17.8% scored positively for eating disorder symptomatology alone,
only 3.1% scored positively for both.

The third research question examined the relationship between problem drinking and specific subscales of the EDI-2. Although the overall
MANOVA was significant, only one subscale was significant, the Impulse Regulation subscale. This result differs from two previous studies
of undergraduate women that found significant relationships between
problem drinking and a number of EDI subscales. One possible explanation may be that the previous studies used the original EDI. The Impulse Regulation subscale is a provisional scale, new to the EDI-2. It
was designed to tap impulsive behaviors, with alcohol abuse among
them.[32] It may be that the new subscale is picking up some of the variance that might have been attributed to other subscales in its absence.
Kashubeck and Mintz[28] indicated that although the relationship with the
various subscales was significant, the difference between groups was
small. It is possible that the Impulse Regulation subscale more accu-
rately captures the relationship between problem drinking and eating
disorder symptomatology. Such a statement must be tentative and made
with extreme caution since such a comparison was not made in the present study. Nonetheless, the results of the present study do lend support
to the validity of the Impulse Regulation subscale since there was a significant relationship with one of the domains it purports to measure.

The final analysis compared women who were members of a sorority
with women who were not sorority members. There was not a significant relationship between sorority membership and eating disorder

status, but there was a significant relationship between sorority membership and problem drinking status, with sorority members more likely to screen positively for problem drinking. This seems to be in contrast to previous studies that have found both problems to be more prevalent among sorority members.[33,34] It appears that in this sample eating disorder symptomatology was rather prevalent among both sorority and non-sorority women, while problem drinking was more prevalent among sorority members than in the general population. It is possible that eating disorder symptomatology is socially acceptable, perhaps even socially encouraged, across a college population, but problem drinking has a narrower range of acceptance. Women may limit their behavior to what they feel is least likely to draw attention to themselves. Once in a situation which allows, supports, or encourages a broader range of behavior, specifically problematic use of alcohol, they may expand their repertoire of symptoms.

In looking at the study overall, there are a number of things to consider. If there are links between chemical dependency and eating disorders as some researchers have suggested,[18-21] it may be worth exploring further the specific nature of that relationship. This study examined co-occurrence and found a very limited relationship. It seems that in this sample there may be a specific sub-population for whom impulsive and destructive behavior manifests itself in both drinking and eating disordered behavior. Factors that could potentially contribute to that may be worth further study.

It is also important to keep in mind that co-occurrence need not be the only way the two are related. Krahn[21] suggested that the coprevalence of these disorders could be manifested in either concurrent or sequential diagnoses. Brisman and Siegel[18] discussed "symptom substitution." In both instances the authors suggested that the two types of problems are so similar that it is easy for a woman who has suffered one to replace it with the other if underlying issues are not resolved. It is important for clinicians to keep this in mind when treating women experiencing either problem. It is also important to do longitudinal studies that could examine if, when, and under what circumstances such symptom substitution occurs.

Finally, it would seem important to consider the possibility that eating disorders may be a way for college women to experience addiction that is more in keeping with the personally destructive but not socially disruptive patterns discussed earlier. If eating disorders and problem drinking are linked, it may be that some college women experience eating disorders *instead* of problem drinking rather than in addition to it.

The prevalence rates of men and women in this study suggest that this might be an area worth exploring, both through research and in clinical practice.

As with any study, this one has its limitations. First, as discussed in the introduction, existing research has found numerous mediating factors related to both problem drinking and eating disorders. This study did not examine them. They warrant further consideration, especially from a perspective that considers the role of gender. Striegel-Moore and Cachelin[5] and Smolak and Murren[35] comment that research on eating disorders seems to be moving away from gender-related considerations and argue for a return to work that examines this. Smolak and Murnen[35] discuss the practice of conceptualizing eating disordered behavior "as primarily individual pathology" and argue for an exploration of sociocultural explanations as well. It seems important to also consider this with respect to problem drinking. Future research and clinical practice need to look more closely at how sociocultural proscriptions regarding gender play themselves out in college students' involvement with alcohol and disordered eating, especially in relation to mediating factors that have already been linked with these problems.

In addition, there are limits to using screening instruments rather than diagnostic procedures. Although screening instruments are appropriate when examining a general population, positive scores primarily suggest the need for more thorough assessment. They do not offer a firm diagnosis and they do not provide a clear picture of what the symptoms mean in a given individual. This is particularly important with respect to eating disorders, which have two primary classifications, anorexia nervosa and bulimia nervosa. A positive score on the EDI-2 is determined by comparing an overall profile to templates provided in the manual. Although subscale elevations may give some indication of anorexia or bulimia, a clinical interview would be required to firmly establish this. Given that in this and previous studies relationships with problem drinking have been linked more to bulimia and impulse regulation than to anorexia, it is possible that lack of co-occurance in this study was due to the nature of eating disorder symptoms present in the positive scores. Thus, there is a need for future research that looks more closely at anorexia and bulimia independently with respect to problem drinking.

Another limitation was the skewed nature of the data. There were far fewer participants who screened positively than negatively for either problem or for all problems combined. Given the nature of the study, a normal distribution would not be expected. Yet, statistically, skewed data can be tricky. It seemed important to respect the integrity of the data and allow them their full range and distribution, however, in so doing, the assumptions of statistical tests were not always completely met.

An effort was made to draw samples that would be representative of a general population of undergraduate women and men, as well as draw from a subpopulation (sorority members) generally considered to be at higher risk for both problem drinking and eating disorders. Nonetheless, this was not a true random sample. This must be considered when attempting to generalize beyond the sample itself. This is particularly important with respect to more diverse populations since this sample was primarily Caucasian.

REFERENCES

1. Brennan AF, Walfish S, AuBuchon P. Alcohol use and abuse in college students. I. A review of individual and personality correlates. Int J Addict. 1986;21:449-474.

2. Capraro RC. Why college men drink: Alcohol, adventure, and the paradox of masculinity. J Am Coll Health. 2000;48:307-315.

3. Engs RC, Hanson DJ. Gender differences in drinking patterns and problems among college students: A review of the literature. J Alcohol Drug Educ. 1990;35: 36-47.

4. Humara MJ, Sherman MF. Statistical determinants of alcohol abuse among Caucasian and African American college students. Addict Behav. 1999;24:135-138.

5. Striegel-Moore RH, Cachelin, FM. Etiology of eating disorders in women. Couns Psychol. 2001;29:635-661.

6. Burns WD, Sloane DC, eds. Students, alcohol, and college health: A special issue (Special Issue). J Am Coll Health. 1987;36:109-110.

7. Ratliff KG, Burkhart BR. Sex differences in motivations for and effects of drinking among college students. J Stud Alcohol. 1984;45:26-32.

8. Wechsler H, Dowdall GW, Davenport A, Rimm EB. A gender-specific measure of binge drinking among college students. Am J Public Health. 1995;85:982-985.

9. Wechsler H, Dowdall GW, Maenner G, et al. Changes in binge drinking and related problems among American college students between 1993 and 1997: Results of the Harvard School of Public Health College Alcohol Study. J Am Coll Health. 1998;47:57-68.

10. O'Hare TM. Drinking in college: Consumption patterns, problems, sex differences, and legal drinking age. J Stud Alcohol. 1990;51:536-541.

11. Perkins HW. Gender patterns in consequences of collegiate alcohol abuse: A 10-year study of trends in an undergraduate population. J Stud Alcohol 1992;53: 458-462.

12. MacDonald R, Fleming MF, Barry KL. Risk factors associated with alcohol abuse in college students. Am J Drug Alcohol Abuse. 1991;17:439-449.

13. Moos RH, Moos BS, Kulik JA. College-student abstainers, moderate drinkers, and heavy drinkers: A comparative analysis. J Youth Adoles. 1976;5:349-369.

14. Reiskin H, Weschler H. Drinking among college students using a campus mental health center. J Stud Alcohol. 1981;42:716-724.

15. Robbins C. Sex differences in psychosocial consequences of alcohol and drug abuse. J Health Soc Behav. 1989;30:117-130.

16. Horowitz AV, White HR. Gender role orientations and styles of pathology among adolescents. J Health Soc Behav. 1987;28:158-170.

17. Oliver JM, Reed CKS, Smith BW. Patterns of psychological problems in university undergraduates: Factor structure of symptoms of anxiety and depression, physical symptoms, alcohol use, and eating problems. Soc Behav Pers. 1998;26:211-232.

18. Brisman J, Siegel M. Bulimia and alcoholism: Two sides of the same coin? J Subst Abuse Treat. 1984;1:113-118.

19. Cooper SE. Chemical dependency and eating disorders: Are they really so different? J Couns Dev. 1989;68:102-105.

20. Gleason NA. College women and alcohol: A relational perspective. J Am Coll Health. 1994;42:279-289.

21. Krahn DD. The relationship of eating disorders and substance abuse. J Subst Abuse. 1991;3:239-253.

22. Sigall BA. The panhellenic task force on eating disorders: A program of primary and secondary prevention for sororities. In: Piran N, Levine MP, Steiner-Adair C, eds. Preventing Eating Disorders: A Handbook of Interventions and Special Challenges. Philadelphia, PA: Bruner/Mazel, 1999:222-237.

23. Greenberg BR. Predictors of binge eating in bulimic and nonbulimic women. Int J Eat Disord. 1986;5:269-284.

24. Pettinati HM, Franks V, Wade JH, Kogan LG. Distinguishing the role of eating disturbance from depression in the sex role self-perceptions of anorexic and bulimic inpatients. J Abnorm Psychol. 1987;96:280-282.

25. Brouwers M. Depressive thought content among female college students with bulimia. J Couns Dev. 1988;66:425-428.

26. Wechsler H, Rohman M, Solomon L. Emotional problems and concerns of New England college students. Am J Orthopsychiatry. 1981;51:719-723.

27. Lundholm JK. Alcohol use among university females: Relationship to eating disordered behavior. Addict Behav. 1989;14:181-185.

28. Kashubeck S, Mintz LB. Eating disorder symptomatology and substance use in college females. J Coll Student Dev. 1996;37:396-404.

29. Babor TF, de la Fuente JR, Saunders J, Grant M. AUDIT, The Alcohol Use Identification Test: Guidelines for use in primary health care. Geneva, Switzerland: World Health Organization, 1989.

30. Saunders JB, AAsland OG, Babor TF, et al. Development of the Alcohol Use Disorders Identification Test (AUDIT): WHO collaborative project on early detection of persons with harmful alcohol consumption–II. Addiction. 1993;88:791-804.

31. Flemming MF, Barry KL, MacDonald R. The alcohol use disorders identification test (AUDIT) in a college sample. Int J Addict. 1991;26:1173-1185.

32. Garner DM. The Eating Disorder Inventory–2: Professional Manual. Odessa, FL: Psychological Assessment Resources, 1991.

33. Meilman PW, von Hippel FA, Gaylor MS. Self-induced vomiting in college women: Its relation to eating, alcohol use, and Greek life. J Am Coll Health. 1991; 40:39-41.

34. Werner MJ, Greene JW. Problem drinking among college freshmen. J Adolesc Health. 1992;13:498-492.

35. Smolak L, Murnen SK. Gender and eating problems. In: Striengel-Moore RH, Smolak L, eds. Eating Disorders: Innovative Directions in Research and Practice. Washington, DC: American Psychological Association, 2001: 91-110.

Genes and/or Jeans?:
Genetic and Socio-Cultural Contributions
to Risk for Eating Disorders

Anne E. Becker, MD, PhD
Pamela Keel, PhD
Eileen P. Anderson-Fye, EdD
Jennifer J. Thomas, BA

SUMMARY. Eating disorders are prevalent among young adult females and pose serious psychological and medical risks. Notwithstanding important advances, efforts to develop effective means of preventing and treating eating disorders have been limited by an incomplete understanding of their multifactorial etiology. Whereas epidemiologic data strongly suggest the influence of socio-cultural context in moderating risk, many hypotheses about how these effects are exerted have remained empirically unevaluated. Specifically, experimental and obser-

Anne E. Becker is affiliated with the Adult Eating and Weight Disorders Program, Department of Psychiatry, Massachusetts General Hospital and the Department of Social Medicine, Harvard Medical School.

Pamela Keel is affiliated with the Department of Psychology, University of Iowa.

Eileen P. Anderson-Fye is affiliated with the Center for Culture and Health, Neuropsychiatric Institute, University of California, Los Angeles.

Jennifer J. Thomas is affiliated with the Department of Psychology, Yale University.

Address correspondence to: Anne E. Becker, MD, PhD, Massachusetts General Hospital–WAC 816, 15 Parkman Street, Boston, MA 02114.

[Haworth co-indexing entry note]: "Genes and/or Jeans?: Genetic and Socio-Cultural Contributions to Risk for Eating Disorders." Becker, Anne E. et al. Co-published simultaneously in *Journal of Addictive Diseases* (The Haworth Medical Press, an imprint of The Haworth Press, Inc.) Vol. 23, No. 3, 2004, pp. 81-103; and: *Eating Disorders, Overeating, and Pathological Attachment to Food: Independent or Addictive Disorders?* (ed: Mark S. Gold) The Haworth Medical Press, an imprint of The Haworth Press, Inc., 2004, pp. 81-103. Single or multiple copies of this article are available for a fee from The Haworth Document Delivery Service [1-800-HAWORTH, 9:00 a.m. - 5:00 p.m. (EST). E-mail address: docdelivery@haworthpress.com].

http://www.haworthpress.com/web/JAD
© 2004 by The Haworth Press, Inc. All rights reserved.
Digital Object Identifer: 10.1300/J069v23n03_07

vational data suggest that social transition (e.g., transnational migration, urbanization, modernization), Western media exposure, and certain peer environments (involving social comparison and teasing) may all contribute to risk. With respect to genetic influences on etiology, family and twin studies have supported a genetic diathesis to eating disorders. Whereas, molecular genetic studies have generated interesting leads–with the most promising findings emerging for genes related to the function of serotonin–they have yet to identify well-replicated susceptibility loci. This paper reviews the data supporting both socio-cultural and genetic contributions for eating disorders and suggests productive future strategies for continuing to unravel their likely multiple and complex interactions. *[Article copies available for a fee from The Haworth Document Delivery Service: 1-800-HAWORTH. E-mail address: <docdelivery@haworthpress. com> Website: <http://www.HaworthPress.com> © 2004 by The Haworth Press, Inc. All rights reserved.]*

KEYWORDS. Genetic, socio-cultural, eating disorders

Eating disorders affect 5 million Americans[1] and pose serious medical and psychological risks. Efforts to identify effective preventive and treatment strategies for eating disorders have been limited by an incomplete understanding of their complex and multifactorial etiology. Rather than embark on a needlessly polarized and presently irresolvable debate concerning relative genetic, psycho-developmental, and socio-cultural contributions to their etiology, we review the robust evidence for *both* socio-cultural and genetic underpinnings of eating disorders and conclude with suggestions for their dialectical relationship to risk. Psycho-developmental contributions to the etiology for eating disorders, for which there is also strong evidence, are beyond the scope of this brief review but likely interface substantially with genetic and socio-cultural factors.

We do not propose a radically socio-cultural view of causal factors, given the presence of clinically significant eating disorders outside of a modern Western context as well as the relatively low base rate of eating disorders within modern Western cultures. Nor do we propose a radically genetic view of causal factors for eating disorders on the basis that concordance for eating disorders in monozygotic twins falls below 1.0. Because neither view provides a complete understanding of etiology, this review follows both lines of research.

EVIDENCE FOR SOCIO-CULTURAL CONTRIBUTIONS TO ETIOLOGY

Observational, epidemiologic, and experimental data provide strong support for the role of socio-cultural contributions to the etiology of eating disorders. The most compelling evidence stems from case and population data that demonstrate that the prevalence of eating disorders varies with historical, social, cultural, and occupational contexts. A variety of hypotheses for relevant socio-cultural factors that would explain this variation have been tested with experimental studies, although some remain unexplored with empirical data.

Case and Population Data

Recent meta-analyses support a significant increase in the incidence of eating disorders during the 20th century[2] suggesting a link to socio-historical context. Cross-cultural data demonstrate variation in the prevalence of eating disorders across diverse social contexts as well. Eating disorders are most prevalent in post-industrial Western nations, though they have been reported virtually around the globe.[2,3] Prevalence rates of eating disorders appear to be consistent across English-speaking North America and Western Europe. In addition, prevalence rates in Eastern Europe and non-Western industrialized societies such as South Korea appear to be on par with or approaching Western rates.[4,5]

A growing number of epidemiologic studies from populations undergoing transnational migration, modernization, or urbanization also underscore the influence of socio-cultural context. For example, several studies have demonstrated that *immigration* into a Western society is associated with elevated risk for disordered eating. Immigrant populations of South Asian girls in Britain,[6] Arab students in London,[7] and Greek women in Munich[8] have been reported to have higher levels of disordered eating than counterparts in their country of origin. An additional study found rates of bulimia nervosa and disordered eating attitudes were even higher among immigrant Pakistani schoolgirls than within the British host population.[9] A rare counter to this pattern was found among women in South Korea who reported significantly more disordered eating attitudes compared with Korean American immigrants to the United States.[10] This latter study indicates need for a finer grained investigation of specific elements of both Western and non-Western social contexts that might increase risk for eating disorders.

In the same vein, a higher prevalence of eating disorders has been found consistently in urban areas compared with rural areas in the cross-cultural record.[11,12] Possibly related, a clear association between *upward mobility* and disordered eating has been observed across diverse cultural settings both among ethnic minority women in the United States,[13,14] ethnic minority women in Britain,[15] and women in modernizing, non-Western societies (e.g., Curaçao, Fiji, South Africa, and Belize).[16-19] Taken together, these data suggest cultural context and/or *social transition* may contribute to risk across diverse ethnic and social groups.

Next, the cultural underpinnings of eating disorders are also suggested by variations in their phenomenology–specifically, in the cultural meanings of and investment in thinness as a goal. For example, the "fear of fatness" presumed to be central to the diagnosis of anorexia nervosa was conspicuously absent in a substantial proportion of Chinese clinic patients diagnosed with the disorder in Hong Kong.[20] Based on this repeated finding,[21] Lee suggests that a "non-fat phobic" subtype of anorexia nervosa exists that is related to but distinct from current Western-based diagnoses. Similarly, data from Indian subjects have suggested absence of characteristic body image disturbance seen in Western subjects[22] as well as a difference in body image constructs.[23] In Belize and in Fiji, disordered eating appears associated with an instrumental concern with attaining a better job, suggesting that disordered eating behavior and body image disturbance may not be universally associated as has been assumed.[17,19] Understanding which aspects of eating disorders vary with social context will help to distinguish sociocultural from genetic and neurophysiologic contributions to risk.

Theoretical Understandings of Socio-Cultural Contributions to Risk

Both historical and cross-cultural evidence strongly suggest that social and cultural contexts are contributors to risk for eating disorders, yet the likely multiple and complex ways in which socio-cultural contexts moderate risk remain incompletely understood. A now classic model for how cultural context promotes risk for disordered eating posits that the cultural valuation of thinness (which prevails in many Western societies) is internalized in some individuals. In vulnerable individuals, this internalized thin ideal leads to body dissatisfaction and, in turn, to disordered eating.[24,25] Vulnerability appears related to gender (with prevalence being universally higher in females), Westernized, post-industrial cultural settings, *social transition (e.g., in immigrant, upwardly mobile*, and modernizing populations), and likely genetic factors (reviewed in the latter sections of this article).

Modernization and social transition are also thought to contribute to risk for eating disorders. In a study in China comparing secondary school students in three communities on a continuum of socioeconomic development, Lee and Lee found increasingly disordered eating attitudes and concern about fatness from the least to the most developed areas.[26] The authors concluded that societal modernization fosters Western-type disordered eating in Chinese women, possibly via the gendered social constraints that accompany it. Not only do structural factors shift with modernization, but also media (with ideas, ideals, and images) and goods saturated with specific messages of the "ideal" thin woman and the malleable body often become more readily available.[27] It appears that acculturative stresses involved in *immigration, upward mobility, or socio-cultural change* may contribute to risk for developing eating disorders independently of Western cultural content. For example, stress related to acculturative processes in the presence of body dissatisfaction was found to place U.S. minority women at greater risk for bulimic symptoms.[28]

The Transitioning Socio-Cultural Context of Gender

One of the most widely discussed theories explaining the association between cultural context and eating disorders has been that the juxtaposition of traditional and modernized gender roles result in conflicts that find expression in eating disorders.[29,30] On the one hand, women in the U.S. have gained increasing social and economic power, while on the other hand the standards for beauty and self-imposed bodily monitoring and discipline have become more stringent. Several researchers have correlated women's increasing educational success and economic power over the latter half of the twentieth century with a reduction in size and curvaceousness of idealized images of women.[24,31] In addition, one small study among American girls suggested an association between attempts to maintain femininity while pursuing achievement and disordered eating.[32] Similarly, cross-cultural data suggest that risk for disordered eating is heightened when alternatives to traditional female roles are introduced through media or migration.[17,33] However, large scale epidemiologic studies have not established a causal link between transitioning gender roles and disordered eating.

Media Influence

Western media images and messages are believed to contribute to the risk for disordered eating.[33,34] However, the specific relationship between individual vulnerability, general cultural values and mores, the failure to represent realistic diversity of (non-slender) body shapes, and the association of thinness with social prestige to risk are as yet unclear. Moreover, it is uncertain whether media simply reflect or create the social preference for slimness, though there is little disagreement that media perpetuate social consensus about ideal body types.[34] Nonetheless, recent experimental and observational data suggest several pathways by which media images and messages have effects on body image and eating disordered behavior. For example, in one experiment with college women, slides of fashion models were found to immediately and negatively impact mood and body satisfaction, two variables thought to be linked with symptoms of disordered eating.[35] Similarly, Stice et al.[36] found a direct linkage between media exposure and disordered eating, with mediational factors of internalization of ideal body type and body satisfaction. Among adolescent girls, attempting to look like the female images in magazines and on television was found to account for variance in weight concerns, though peer emphasis on weight was even more important.[37] One innovative study found that it was not the frequency but rather the content of television viewed that impacted body dissatisfaction.[38] Media exposure also has been shown to elicit different responses from women with and without eating disorders, further supporting the hypothesis that the images play some pathogenic role in perpetuating the disorders among vulnerable individuals.[39,40] Such data all strongly suggest that internalization of certain types of female images impact body dissatisfaction and eating disordered symptoms.

Of note, not all studies have been able to discern clear impact of media exposure on disordered eating.[41] One of the likely methodologic limitations of investigating the relationship between media consumption and disordered eating stems from the saturation of media exposure in Western populations, which are chronically and nearly universally exposed. Therefore, additional compelling data on the pathogenic effects of media on the development of eating disordered attitudes and behaviors comes from studying the emergence of disordered eating in cultural contexts in which Western media images and messages are newly introduced. For instance, the introduction of Western television to rural Fiji was associated with an increase in disordered eating attitudes and behaviors among adolescent girls there. Changes were especially dramatic and salient given that traditional Fijian culture valued robust body size and appetites and eating disorders were believed to be rare or non-existent in the indigenous population prior to the introduction of television.[17] Moreover, qualitative data showed that girls aspired to the social and material trappings of affluent Western lifestyles depicted on television which they associated with thinness. In this setting of rapid social change, television programming not only transmitted images that supported the social value of thinness but also promoted weight control as a legitimate means of positioning oneself competitively vis a vis peers.

Peer Influence, Teasing, and Social Comparison

Peer relations are another domain of social context apparently important to risk for development of eating disorders. Paxton et al.[42] found eating attitudes to be similar within friendship cliques among adolescent girls, and moreover, that an individual's extreme weight loss behaviors could be predicted by the behaviors among her friends. Extending this work, Meyer and Waller[43] found that restrictive eating and body concerns (socially valued attitudes) increased over time among women with social proximity in apartment buildings, while bulimic attitudes (not socially valued) diverged. It follows that spending time in sub-cultural contexts in which peers emphasize thinness and dietary restraint contributes to risk for the development of eating disorders. In a study of 523 grade school and middle school students, the emphasis peers put on weight and eating was found to be the most important predictor of weight-related concerns.[44] Similarly, Crandall found that binge-eating in individuals in a sorority was predicted by the level of binge-eating among friends and that the closer the friendship became, the more similar the level of binge-eating became.[45] Finally, the higher prevalence of eating disorders in occupational groups where thinness or leanness is valued such as models, actors, dancers, gymnasts, figure skaters, rowers, wrestlers, and jockeys[3,46] supports the role of social pressures in moderating risk.

Several studies have drawn on social comparison theory[47] in order to explain mediating factors of how those with eating disorders internalize messages from teasing[48] or the media.[49] Those who evaluate themselves in comparison to media images have been found to have more eating disorder symptomatology and higher body image dissatisfaction than those who do not. Among female undergraduates, social comparison was found to be a significant predictor of body dissatisfaction and eating disturbance,[50] particularly when the target of comparison was subjectively important.[51] Further, Thompson et al.[48] found appearance-based social comparison to mediate the effect of appearance-related teasing on body image and eating disturbance. Interestingly, among high school aged girls, those who evaluated self-esteem based on close relationships (e.g., as opposed to achievement-based evaluations) were more likely to report eating disorder symptoms and higher body dissatisfaction than other girls.[52] Because ideas and images transmitted through the media are primary cultural resources from which adolescents draw to establish peer norms and ideals, further research is required to understand the relative and likely synergistic roles of peer-generated social pressure and peer-group media exposure.

Teasing is an important means by which peer influence is exerted and reinforced. Because teasing presumably highlights and implicitly criticizes discrepancies between actual and ideal attributes or behaviors according to social norms, it is not surprisingly associated with disordered eating attitudes and behaviors.[53] Among overweight adolescents, binge-eating was significantly associated with weight-related teasing for both girls and boys.[82] Similarly, a longitudinal study of adolescent girls found a teasing history to be significantly related to the development of body image and eating disturbance for both obese and non-obese subjects at three-year follow-up.[54] Moreover, another study identified teasing as a partial mediator between BMI and dietary restraint among adolescent girls in Sweden and Australia.[55] Finally, among women with BED, appearance-based teasing history was related to higher body dissatisfaction.[56]

Conclusions About Socio-Cultural Contributions to Risk for Eating Disorders

In summary, the historical, geographical, and cultural distribution of eating disorders strongly suggests that specific features of socio-cultural context moderate risk, though the exact mechanisms through which this occurs are still not well understood. Based on the available evidence, it is highly likely that socio-cultural dynamics associated with post-industrialization, modernization, and Western cultural features contribute to social environments which, in some way, support disordered eating and body image disturbance. However, specific pathogenic elements of Western and post-industrialized societies still remain mostly empirically unevaluated. Hypotheses based upon clinical and sociological observational data include conflict over transitioning gender-appropriate roles for women, the association of thinness with social value (promoted in part through the media), and the importance of body shape in competitive social positioning as cultural elements that may increase risk. These may partially explain presently emerging population data linking social transition to risk for disordered eating. Finally, within a population, it appears there is empirical support that peer environment (e.g., emphasis on social comparison and prevalence and content of teasing) as well as media exposure may play an important role in moderating risk for the development of eating disorders as well.

The salience of environmental contributions to complex diseases has been best demonstrated with changes in prevalence of illness when populations migrate from countries with low-risk to high-risk. Similarly, they are suggested by changes in disease rates in one population over time–presumably as socio-cultural factors support environmental risk factors.[57] Thus, the emerging population data that demonstrate the link between migration and modernization and increased prevalence in eating disorders strongly support an environmental contribution to risk. Opportunities to isolate and investigate suspected social risk factors for eating disorders will be a critical component to future research. Indeed, the rapid social change in many developing societies resulting from globalization presents an opportunity to understand (and possibly to intervene in) the pathogenesis of eating disorders.

EVIDENCE FOR GENETIC CONTRIBUTIONS TO ETIOLOGY

There are several compelling lines of evidence to suggest a genetic contribution to the pathogenesis of eating disorders. Similar to many other forms of psychopathology, eating disorders cluster in families. In addition, twin studies routinely yield substantial heritability estimates. However, the hunt for genetic susceptibility loci–while showing some promising leads–has generated more questions than answers.

Behavioral Genetic Research

Recent studies suggest that biological relatives of eating disorder probands incur a 5 to 12-fold increase in risk of developing an eating disorder.[58-60] The marked familial aggregation[60] with effects diminishing from first to third degree relatives[59] is consistent with models of genetic clustering. However, it is not possible to disentangle the effects of genes and environment on these observed patterns as family members generally share both. In order to differentiate the influence of genes from the influence of environment, twin studies have been conducted.

Studies examining eating disorder concordance among members of population-based twin registries in Virginia, Minnesota, Australia, and Denmark point toward a sizeable genetic component. Investigators have determined anorexia nervosa to be highly heritable, with genes accounting for 58% to 76%[61] of the variance in morbidity. Data on bulimia nervosa have been more variable, with heritability estimates ranging from 30%[62] to 83%.[63] However, much of this variation appears to be related to problems in diagnostic reliability. That is, in a simple additive model, variability due to error (such as lack of agreement in diagnosing a disorder) inflates the estimated contribution of non-shared environment and could result in an underestimate of genetic or shared environmental effects.[64] Bulik et al. reported a particularly high estimate of heritability for bulimia nervosa (83%) when using a highly reliable assessment.[63] Genes also have been implicated in explaining a similar proportion of the variance in attitudes[65,66] and behaviors[67] characteristic of disordered eating.

Despite the plethora of studies indicating that eating disorders may be as heritable as schizophrenia or bipolar disorder, the results should be examined with care given the nature of these disorders. Violations of both the Equal Environments and Representativeness assumptions have been proposed to conflate heritability estimates for eating disorders.[64] The first assumption, that the shared environment of monozygotic twin pairs is not more similar than the shared environment of dizygotic twins is frequently invalid. For example, Hettema et al. found physical similarity[68] and Kendler and Gardner found degree of cosocialization[69] to be significantly greater in monozygotic compared to dizygotic twins and to be significant predictors of bulimia nervosa concordance in twins. However, Klump et al. found that neither general physical similarity nor body size/shape similarity was significantly associated with twin similarity for eating attitudes and behaviors.[70] Aside from physical similarity, Fichter and Noegel point out that being a member of a twin pair, particularly a monozygotic twin pair, may be a risk factor for disordered eating by limiting the development of an autonomous self,[71] and Waters et al. noted differential clinical presentations between eating disordered twins and singletons.[72] These authors suggested that twins may be not representative of the general population when attempting to understand the etiology of eating disorders. However, studies utilizing larger, population-based twin samples have found that twins and non-twins were at equal risk for several different types of psychopathology, including eating disorders.[73,74] Thus, although violations of the Equal Environments and Representativeness assumptions could inflate heritability estimates for eating disorders, these violations do not fully account for the greater similarity in eating disorders between monozygotic compared to dizygotic twins.

In summary, behavioral genetic studies provide compelling evidence of a genetic contribution to eating disorders, but they do not reveal specific genes exerting this influence. Following advances in human genome mapping, an exciting avenue of research examines specific genetic loci associated with increased risk for eating disorders.

Molecular Genetic Studies

Unlike results from family and twin studies, well-replicated results have yet to emerge from studies examining the specific genes that are believed to confer risk for developing an eating disorder. Most molecular genetic research has involved association studies in which the frequency of alleles for specific genes or gene markers ("candidate genes") are compared between individuals affected with a disorder and those unaffected. Alternatively, the frequency of allele transmission from heterozygous parents to affected offspring is compared to that expected if there is no association between the allele and disorder (transmission disequilibrium test; TDT). A third approach involves a genome-wide linkage analysis evaluating alleles at several genetic markers that are shared by affected relatives at a greater frequency than would be expected by chance. These approaches have produced a number of interesting leads.

Candidate Gene Studies

Given the role of serotonin in regulating satiety,[75] mood,[76] and impulse control[77] and the efficacy of selective serotonin reuptake inhibitors in treating bulimia nervosa, genes that impact serotonin function represent prime candidates for understanding the genetic etiology of eating disorders. Five reports have found an association between anorexia nervosa and elevated frequency of the A allele and A/A genotype of the 5-HT_{2A} receptor–1438 gene.[78-82] However, five other studies have failed to replicate this finding[83-87] among anorexic, bulimic, or obese populations. Similarly, meta-analyses of the 5-HT_{2A} data have yielded conflicting findings. Two meta-analyses have supported an association between the 5-HT_{2A} receptor gene and anorexia nervosa (Kipman et al.[86] and Collier et al.[88]), and one meta-analysis has not supported this association (Ziegler et al.[87]). Pieri and Campbell suggested that meta-analyses have been uninformative because the genetic endowment of control groups has differed significantly across studies.[89] Thus, inconsistent results could be due to the effect of genetically different control groups when calculating odds ratios for allele transmission to patients with anorexia nervosa. Similar to differences in control populations, substantial differences in eating disorder phenotypes may account for inconsistent findings. For example, three studies[80-82] have suggested that the A allele and A/A genotype for the $5\text{-HT}_{2A}-1438$ gene are elevated in the restricting subtype of anorexia nervosa and not the binge-purge subtype, and one study found an association between bulimic symptoms and the G allele.[90] Moreover, valid phenotypic differences may not be captured by the current diagnostic criteria for eating disorders.

No other candidate genes have produced findings to equal those associated with the 5-HT_{2A} receptor. Of interest, two studies have reported an association between the estrogen beta receptor gene and anorexia nervosa.[91,92] This result may explain observed developmental changes in heritability for disordered eating attitudes and behaviors. Klump et al. observed greater genetic influence on eating attitudes and behaviors in 17-year-old twins compared to 11-year-old twins.[93] In a subsequent investigation, Klump et al. reported increased heritability of disordered eating in post-pubertal compared to pre-pubertal 11-year old twins, concluding that the time-release effects of estrogen may contribute to the usually post-pubertal presentation of disordered eating.[94]

Candidate Gene Studies Using Transmission Disequilibrium Tests

One study utilizing Transmission Disequilibrium Tests (TDTs) to assess transmission of the A and G alleles of the 5-HT_{2A} receptor–1438 gene found no significant result.[95] However, a follow-up investigation analyzing a subset of patients with a later age of onset (mean age = 15 years) demonstrated increased transmission of the $5\text{-HT}_{2A}-1438$ A allele.[86] Kipman et al. suggested that previous replication problems in candidate gene studies might be due to differences in the age of patient sample examined. Further, these results suggest that age of onset may serve as a potential feature for making phenotypic distinctions that is not recognized in current diagnostic systems. Conversely, Kipman et al. failed to find a difference between the restricting and purging subtypes of anorexia nervosa for this candidate gene. Most TDT studies of other candidate genes have not reported significant findings for eating disorders. Exceptions to this pattern include a study by Frisch et al.[96] indicating increased transmission of the H allele of the COMT Val/Met 158 gene and a study by Koronyo-Hamaoui et al.[97] demonstrating increased transmission of longer CAG repeats of the hSKCa3 potassium channel gene to patients with anorexia nervosa. Both results require replication in future studies.

Genome-Wide Linkage Analyses

A genome-wide linkage analysis demonstrated a modest peak reflecting alleles shared above chance on chromosome 4 for anorexia nervosa probands and their eating disordered relatives. However, when analyses were restricted to families sharing the restricting subtype of anorexia nervosa, a significant peak was reported on chromosome one.[98] Similarly, a genome-wide linkage analysis of bulimia nervosa probands and their eating disorder relatives in which all individuals engaged in self-induced vomiting found a peak on chromosome 10p.[99]

Overall, the most promising findings have emerged for genes related to the function of serotonin. Although association analyses are theoretically informed and have yielded interesting results, they represent a somewhat limited approach for exploring potential genetic loci in comparison to genome-wide linkage analyses. That is, association analyses rely on a good working knowledge of the biological antecedents (versus consequences) of eating disorders in order to identify candidate genes. Given the uncertain pathogenesis of eating disorders, it is difficult to disentangle such factors. As can be seen from Table 1, most molecular genetic studies have investigated anorexia nervosa and not bulimia nervosa or binge-eating disorder. Thus, in addition to further research on the genetic bases of eating disorders, this work would benefit from examination of different eating disorder subtypes, both as defined within the current nosological systems as well as by new approaches to identify valid phenotypes. Results from a recent review of the epidemiological, cross-historical, and cross-cultural data for anorexia nervosa and bulimia nervosa suggest that these may be etiologically distinct syndromes.[2] Results from some recent molecular genetic studies support this conclusion[2,80,81,99] and suggest that identification of genetic susceptibility loci requires further definition of eating disorder phenotypes.

Conclusions About Genetic Contributions to Risk for Eating Disorders

Whereas behavioral genetic studies have supported a genetic diathesis to eating disorders, molecular genetic studies have yet to identify well-

TABLE 1. Candidate Gene Studies Evaluating Serotonin

Study	Comparison Groups (n)	Target Polymorphism	Evidence of Association
Collier et al. (1997) [78]	AN (81) > Controls (226)	5-HT$_{2A}$: −1438A and A/A	Yes
Enoch et al. (1998)[79]	AN (88) > BN (59), Controls (213)	5-HT$_{2A}$: −1438A and A/A	Yes
Sorbi et al. (1998)[80]	AN-R (43) > AN-P (34), Controls (107)	5-HT$_{2A}$: −1438A and A/A	Yes
Nacimas et al. (1999)[81]	AN-R (57) > AN-P (52), BN-P (59), Controls (107)	5-HT$_{2A}$: −1438A and A/A, 102TC	Yes
		5-HT$_{2A}$: Thr25Asn; His452Tyr; 516C/T	No
		5-HT2C: Cys-23Ser	No
Nishiguchi et al. (2001)[90]	ED-B+ [AN-B, BN] (136) > ED-B− [AN-R] (36), Controls (374)	5-HT$_{2A}$: −1438G	Yes
Kipman et al. (2002)[86]	AN (145), Controls (98)	5-HT$_{2A}$: −1438A	No
	AN (Mean age at onset = 15.28) > AN (Mean age at onset = 14.01)	5-HT$_{2A}$: −1438A	Yes
Ricca et al. (2002)[82]	Obese BED (54), Obese non-BED (132), Controls (115)	5-HT$_{2A}$: −1438A/G	No
	AN (148), AN-R (74), BN (86) > Controls (115)	5-HT$_{2A}$: −1438 A and A/A	Yes
	AN-P (74), Controls (115)	5-HT$_{2A}$: −1438A/G	No
Hinney et al. (1997)[83]	AN (100), Obese Controls (254), Underweight Controls (101)	5-HT$_{2A}$: −1438 G/A; Thr25Asn; His452Tyr	No
Campbell et al. (1998)[84]	AN (152), Controls (150)	5-HT$_{2A}$: −1438G/A	No
Karwautz et al. (2001)[85]	AN (45), Unaffected Sisters (45)	5-HT$_{2A}$: −1438G/A; 5-HT$_{2C}$: Cys-23Ser	No
Ziegler et al. (1999)[87]	AN (78), BN (99), Controls (170)	5-HT$_{2A}$: −1438G/A	No

Note: A/A, A/G, G/G and s/s, s/l, l/l reflect genotype frequency analyses. A, G, s, or l reflect allele frequency analyses. Subtype designations reflect those used by the original authors, and are not necessarily standardized according to DSM-IV criteria. Participants in Nacimas et al. (1999)[81] are included in Ricca et al. (2002).[82]

replicated susceptibility loci. This degree of progress is likely a reflection of the early stage of molecular genetic research in this area as well as the etiologic complexity of these disorders. As with most psychiatric disorders, the genetic diathesis to eating disorders is likely to involve complex inheritance rather than Mendelian inheritance.[100] This conclusion is supported by two epidemiological patterns. First, eating disorders are associated with a higher prevalence than typical Mendelian diseases. Second, the risk to first-degree relatives (5 to 12-fold) is far below that expected in Mendelian diseases with a dominant gene with complete penetrance (5,000-fold) or a recessive gene with complete penetrance (2,500-fold). Although reduced penetrance (i.e., genotype does not lead to phenotype), variable expressivity (i.e., genotype leads to variable phenotypes), and phenocopies (i.e., phenotype occurs in the absence of genotype) diminish risk ratios for Mendelian diseases, the ratios for Mendelian diseases remain well above those reported for most psychiatric disorders, including eating disorders. Failures to replicate findings likely reflect problems in statistical power when evaluating disorders with complex inheritance in which genotypic relative risks will be modest.[101] Association studies employing candidate genes and TDT have greater power; however, they require tentative identification of the gene and its polymophisms to be tested. An additional challenge in the search for genetic susceptibility loci is the lack of eating disorder phenotypes associated with longitudinal stability.[102] Thus, more research on the nosologic categories of eating disorders is necessary in order to identify valid and reliable phenotypes. Better nosologic characterization will, in turn, allow more efficient progress toward establishing the genetic underpinnings of eating disorders.

CONCLUSIONS

We conclude with a few humble observations about the state of empirical support for genetic and environmental contributions to risk for eating disorders. First, like most psychiatric disorders,[103] eating disorders are clearly complex with both genetic and environmental etiologic components. The respective contributions of each of these components are, at best, only incompletely understood. Second, we are evidently quite far off from grasping the complicated ways in which environment and genes are likely to interact to impact on susceptibility and phenotypic expression. Third, there are multiple methodologic and theoretical challenges to the investigation of both genetic and environmental contributors to risk. These include, the far greater prevalence of disordered eating attitudes and behaviors than clinically significant or syndrome level disorders, the phenotypic heterogeneity of even full-syndrome eating disorders, the substantial crossover between even apparently nosologically distinct eating disorders, and then the myriad of social, cultural, developmental, psychological, and physiologic effects on body image, body habitus, and dietary patterns.

Our understanding of environmental contributions to eating disorders is only rudimentary. In this review, we have focused on environmental factors that stem from socio-cultural factors (really only one component of environmental influences that would also include various psychological and developmental dimensions). The classic hypotheses for how socio-cultural context might contribute to risk have presented major methodologic challenges, given the difficulty of isolating suspected contributors to risk from a socio-cultural matrix in experimental and observational studies. Moreover, some of the hypotheses are based on social analyses and reasonable conjecture, but have not been empirically evaluated.

Similarly, despite impressive progress and enthusiasm in the scientific community genetic contributions to risk can be described only in general terms. That is, twin studies have yielded impressive heritability estimates, but the search for candidate genes has yielded mostly inconsistent data or negative studies to data. A major methodologic challenge in investigating the genetic underpinnings of eating disorders include the phenotypic heterogeneity of these disorders. Thus, our understanding of the complex risk factors that may be transmitted genetically is rudimentary but does show some promising leads.

As Willett has persuasively argued, the most effective interventions for complex diseases will require better integration of both genetic and epidemiologic studies.[57] Moreover, illnesses with heritability patterns which do not follow Mendelian genetics are most likely the end result of genetically mediated vulnerability to a variety of environmental factors.[104] For instance, population data strongly support environmental contributions to risk for disordered eating, but vulnerability of certain individuals within such populations and familial vulnerability is best explained by complex genetic factors that have yet to be specified. Because genes mediating vulnerability likely have their own genetic and environmental modifiers, understanding their relative and interactive contributions to illness enters into "another order of complexity."[104] That is, there are likely gene-gene interactions and gene-environment interactions as well as environment-environment interactions that increase or diminish risk.

Given the complementarity of both genetic and socio-cultural vulnerability factors, new research avenues integrating these approaches should be sought. For example, a traditional family study design applied to United States immigrants could reveal how familial factors might increase vulnerability to acculturative stress. Similarly, twin studies could estimate the relative influence of genetic and environmental factors within transitioning societies where there is still substantial variability in social pressures to be thin. Moreover, epidemiologic studies may identify sources of phenotypic variation across diverse social contexts that will inform genetic studies. These represent just a few possibilities within a myriad of productive collaborations that can emerge from a dialectical approach between genetic and socio-cultural perspectives.

In summary, our efforts to develop effective models for the primary prevention of eating disorders have been disappointing to date,[105] largely due to our incomplete grasp of their complex etiology. In addition, despite many important advances in the treatment of eating disorders, up to 50% of cases of both bulimia and anorexia nervosa follow a chronic course.[106,107] For these reasons, continued efforts to discern how environmental and genetic factors interact to contribute to risk are critical. An integrative approach will ideally utilize strong cross-disciplinary collaboration among clinicians and researchers from the fields of psychiatry, psychology, sociology, anthropology, molecular biology, and genetics, among others, to leverage their relative strengths. We are optimistic that such an approach will be successful in better characterizing the etiology of eating disorders and integrating these findings into ever more effective preventive and therapeutic strategies.

REFERENCES

1. National Institute of Mental Health. Eating Disorders. NIH Publication No. 94-3477. Rockville, MD, 1994.

2. Keel PK, Klump KL. Are eating disorders culture-bound syndromes? Implications for conceptualizing their etiology. Psychol Bull 2003; 129(5):747-69.

3. Anderson-Fye EP, Becker AE. Cultural Aspects of Eating Disorders Across Cultures. The Handbook of Eating Disorders and Obesity, 2003; pp. 565-89, London: Wiley.

4. Boyadjieva S, Steinhausen HC. The Eating Attitudes Test and the Eating Disorders Inventory in four Bulgarian clinical and nonclinical samples. Int J Eat Disord. 1996;19:93-8.

98   *Eating Disorders, Overeating, and Pathological Attachment to Food*

5. Lee YH, Rhee MK, Park SH, et al. Epidemiology of eating disordered symptoms in the Korean general population using a Korean version of the Eating Attitudes Test. Eat Weight Disord. 1998; 3:153-61.

6. Mumford D, Whitehouse A, Choudry I. Survey of eating disorders in English-medium schools in Lahore, Pakistan. Int J Eat Disord. 1992; 11:173-84.

7. Nasser, M. Comparative study of the prevalence of abnormal eating attitudes among Arab female students of both London and Cairo universities. Psychol Med. 1986; 16:621-5.

8. Fichter M, Weyerer S, Sourdi L, Sourdi Z. The epidemiology of anorexia nervosa: A comparison of Greek adolescents living in Germany and Greek adolescents living in Greece. In: Darby PL, Garfinkel PE, Garner DM, Coscina DV (eds.). Anorexia Nervosa: Recent Developments in Research. New York: Alan R. Liss, 1983: 95-105.

9. Mumford DB, Whitehouse AM, Platts M. Sociocultural correlates of eating disorders among Asian schoolgirls in Bradford. Br J Psychiatry. 1991;158:222-8.

10. Ko C, Cohen H. Intraethnic comparison of eating attitudes in native Koreans and Korean Americans using a Korean translation of the eating attitudes test. J Nerv Ment Dis. 1998;186:631-6.

11. Hoek HW, Bartelds AI, Bosveld JJ, et al. Impact of urbanization on detection rates of eating disorders. Am J Psychiatry. 1995;152:1272-8.

12. Kuboki T, Nomura S, Ide M, et al. Epidemiological data on anorexia nervosa in Japan. Psychiatry Res. 1996;62:11-6.

13. Silber TJ. Anorexia nervosa in blacks and Hispanics. Int J Eat Disord. 1986; 5:121-8.

14. Yates A. Current perspectives on the eating disorders: I. History, psychological and biological aspects. J Am Acad Child Adolesc Psychiatry. 1989;28:813-28.

15. Soomro GM, Crisp AH, Lynch D, et al. Anorexia nervosa in 'non-white' populations. Br J Psychiatry. 1995;167:385-9.

16. Hoek H. The occurrence of eating disorders at Curacao. Academy for Eating Disorders International Conference on Eating Disorders. 2002; Boston, MA. Plenary presentation.

17. Becker A, Burwell R, Gilman S, et al. Disordered eating behaviors and attitudes follow prolonged exposure to television among ethnic Fijian adolescent girls. Br J Psychiatry. 2002;180:509-14.

18. Le Grange D, Telch CF, Tibbs J. Eating attitudes and behaviors in 1,435 South African caucasian and non-caucasian college students. Am J Psychiatry. 1998;155: 250-44.

19. Anderson-Fye EP. A Coca-Cola shape: Cultural change, body image, and eating concerns in Belize. Cult Med Psychiatry, In press.

20. Lee S, Ho TP, Hsu LKG. Fat phobic and non-fat phobic anorexia nervosa: A comparative study of 70 Chinese patients in Hong Kong. Psychol Med. 1993;3: 999-1017.

21. Lee S. Self-starvation in context: Towards a culturally sensitive understanding of anorexia nervosa. Soc Sci Medicine. 1995;41:25-36.

22. Khandelwal SK, Sharan P, Saxena S. Eating disorders: An Indian perspective. Int J Soc Psychiatry. 1995;41:132-46.

23. Gupta MA, Chaturvedi SK, Chandarana PC, Johnson AM. Weight-related body image concerns among 18-24 year-old women in Canada and India: An empirical comparative study. J Psychosom Res. 2001;50:193-8.

24. Garner DM, Garfinkel PE. Socio-cultural factors in the development of anorexia nervosa. Psychol Med. 1980;10:647-56.

25. Striegel-Moore RH, Silberstein LR, Rodin J. Toward an understanding of risk factors for bulimia. American Psychologist. 1986;41:246-63.

26. Lee S, Lee AM. Disordered eating in three communities of China: A comparative study of female high school students in Hong Kong, Shenzhen, and rural Hunan. Int J Eat Disord. 2000; 27:317-27.

27. Bordo, S. Unbearable Weight: Feminism, Western Culture, and the Body. Berkeley, CA: University of California, 1993.

28. Perez M, Voelz GL, Pettit JW, Joiner TE. The role of acculturative stress and body dissatisfaction in predicting bulimic symptomatology across ethnic groups. Int J Eat Disord. 2002;32:219-24.

29. Bruch H. Anorexia nervosa and its differential diagnosis. J Nerv Ment Dis. 1966;141:555-66.

30. Perlick D, Silverstein B. Faces of female discontent: Depression, disordered eating, and changing gender roles. In: Fallon PF, Katzman M, Wooley S. (eds.) Feminist Perspectives on Eating Disorders. New York: Guilford Press, 1994:77-93.

31. Barber N. The slender ideal and eating disorders: An interdisciplinary "telescope" model. Int J Eat Disord. 1998;23:295-307.

32. Steiner-Adair, C. The body politic: Normal female adolescent development and the development of eating disorders. In: Gilligan C, Lyons N, Hamner T (eds.). Making Connections: The Relational Worlds of Adolescent Girls at Emma Willard School. Cambridge, MA: Harvard University Press, 1990:162-82.

33. Nasser M. Screening for abnormal eating attitudes in a population of Egyptian secondary school girls. Soc Psychiatry Psychiatr Epidemiol. 1994;29:25-30.

34. Becker AE, Hamburg P. Culture, the media, and eating disorders. Harv Rev Psychiatry. 1996;4:163-7.

35. Pinhas L, Toner BB, Ali A, et al. The effects of the ideal of female beauty on mood and body satisfaction. Int J Eat Disord. 1999;25:223-6.

36. Stice E, Schupak-Neuberg E, Shaw HE, Stein RI. Relation of media exposure to eating disorder symptomatology: An examination of mediating mechanisms. J Abnorm Psychol. 1994;103:836-40.

37. Taylor CB, Sharpe T, Shisslak C, et al. Factors associated with weight concerns in adolescent girls. Int J Eat Disord. 1998;24:31-42.

38. Tiggemann M, Pickering AS. Role of television in adolescent women's body dissatisfaction and drive for thinness. Int J Eat Disord. 1996;20:199-203.

39. Toro J, Salamero M, Martinez E. Assessment of sociocultural influences on the aesthetic body shape model in anorexia nervosa. Acta Psych Scand. 1994;89:147-51.

40. Hamilton K, Waller G. Media influences on body size estimation in anorexia and bulimia. An experimental study. Br J Psychiatry. 1993;162:837-40.

41. Cusumano DL, Thompson JK. Body image and body shape ideals in magazines: Exposure, awareness, and internalization. Sex Roles. 1997;37:701-21.

42. Paxton SJ, Schutz HK, Wertheim EH, Muir SL. Friendship clique and peer influences on body image concerns, dietary restraint, extreme weight-loss behaviors, and binge eating in adolescent girls. J Abnorm Psychol 1999;108:255-66.

43. Meyer C, Waller G. Social convergence of disturbed eating attitudes in young adult women. J Nerv Ment Dis 2001;189:114-19.

44. Taylor CB, Sharpe T, Shisslak C, et al. Factors associated with weight concerns in adolescent girls. Int J Eat Disord 1998;24:31-42.

45. Crandall CS. Social contagion of binge eating. Journal of Personality & Social Psychology. 1988;55:588-98.

46. Sundgot-Borgen, J. Eating disorders among male and female elite athletes. B J Sports Med. 1999; 33:434.

47. Festinger L. A theory of social comparison process. Human Relations 1954; 7:117-40.

48. Thompson JK, Coovert MD, Stormer SM. Body image, social comparison, and eating disturbance: A covariance structure modeling investigation. Int J Eat Disord 1999;26:43-51.

49. Hamilton K, Waller G. Media influences on body size estimation in anorexia and bulimia. An experimental study. Br J Psychiatry 1993;162:837-40.

50. Stormer SM, Thompson JK. Explanations of body image disturbance: A test of maturational status, negative verbal commentary, social comparison, and sociocultural hypotheses. Int J Eat Disord 1996;19:193-202.

51. Thompson JK, Heinberg LJ. Preliminary test of two hypotheses of body image disturbance. Int J Eat Disord 1993;14:59-63.

52. Geller J, Zaitsoff SL, Srikameswaran S. Beyond shape and weight: Exploring the relationship between nonbody determinants of self-esteem and eating disorder symptoms in adolescent females. Int J Eat Disord 2002;32:344-51.

53. Neumark-Sztainer D, Falkner N, Story M, et al. Weight-teasing among adolescents: Correlations with weight status and disordered eating behaviors. International Journal of Obesity 2002;26:123-31.

54. Thompson JK, Coovert MD, Richards KJ, et al. Development of body image, eating disturbance, and general psychological functioning in female adolescents: Covariance structure modeling and longitudinal investigations. Int J Eat Disord 1995; 18:221-36.

55. Lunner K, Werthem EH, Thompson JK, et al. A cross-cultural examination of weight-related teasing, body image, and eating disturbance in Swedish and Australian samples. Int J Eat Disord 2000;28:430-5.

56. Jackson TD, Grilo CM, Masheb RM. Teasing history, onset of obesity, current eating disorder psychopathology, body dissatisfaction, and psychological functioning in binge eating disorder. Obes Res 2000; 8:451-8.

57. Willett WC. Balancing life-style and genomics: Research for disease prevention. Science. 2002;296:695-98.

58. Lilenfield LR, Kaye WH, Greeno G, et al. A controlled family study of anorexia nervosa and bulimia nervosa: Psychiatric disorders in first-degree relatives and effects of proband comorbidity. Arch Gen Psychiatry. 1998;55:603-10.

59. Woodside DB, Field LL, Garfinkel PE, Heinmaa M. Specificity of eating disorders diagnosis in families of probands with anorexia nervosa and bulimia nervosa. Compr Psychiatry. 1998;39:261-64.

60. Strober M, Freeman R, Lampert C, et al. Controlled family study of anorexia nervosa and bulimia nervosa: Evidence of shared liability and transmission of partial syndromes. Am J Psychiatry. 2000;157:393-401.

61. Klump KL, Miller KB, Keel PK, et al. Genetic and environmental influence on anorexia nervosa syndromes in a population-based twin sample. Psychol Med. 2001; 31:737-40.

62. Kendler KS, Walters EE, Neale MC, et al. The structure of the genetic and environmental risk factors for six major psychiatric disorders in women: Phobia, generalized anxiety disorder, panic disorder, bulimia, major depression, and alcoholism. Arch Gen Psychiatry. 1995;52:374-83.

63. Bulik CM, Sullivan PF, Kendler KS. Heritability of binge-eating and broadly defined bulimia nervosa. Biol Psychiatry. 1998;44:1210-18.

64. Plomin R, DeFries JC, McClearn GE, McGuffin P. Behavior Genetics, 4th Edition. Ed Worth: New York, 2001.

65. Wade T, Martin NG, Neale MC, et al. The structure of genetic and environmental risk factors for three measures of disordered eating. Psychol Med. 1999;29:925-34.

66. Rutherford J, McGuffin P, Katz RJ, Murray RM. Genetic influences on eating attitudes in a normal female twin population. Psychol Med. 1993;23:425-36.

67. Sullivan PF, Bulik CM, Kendler KS. Genetic epidemiology of binging and vomiting. Brit J Psychiatry. 1998;173:75-79.

68. Hettema JM, Neale MC, Kendler KS. Physical similarity and the equal environment assumption in twin studies of psychiatric disorders. Behavior Genetics. 1995; 25:327-35.

69. Kendler KS, Gardner CO. Twin studies of adult psychiatric and substance dependence disorders: Are they biased by differences in the environmental experiences of monozygotic and dizygotic twins in childhood and adolescence? Psychol Med. 1998; 28:625-33.

70. Klump KL, Iacono HA, McGue M, Willson LE. Physical similarity and twin resemblence for eating attitudes and behaviors: A test of the equal environment assumption. Behavior Genetics. 2000;30:51-8.

71. Fichter MM, Noegel R. Concordance for bulimia nervosa in twins. Int J Eat Disord 1990;9:255-63.

72. Waters BGH, Beumont PJV, Touyz S, Kennedy M. Behavioural differences between twin and non-twin female sibling pairs discordant for anorexia nervosa. Int J Eat Disord. 1990;9:265-73.

73. Klump KL, Kaye WH, Strober M. The evolving genetic foundations of eating disorders. Psychiatr Clin N Am. 2001;24:215-25.

74. Kendler KS, Martin NG, Heath AC, Eaves LJ. Self-report psychiatric symptoms in twins and their non-twin relatives: Are twins different? Am J Med Genet. 1995;60:588-91.

75. Brewerton TD, Murphy DL, Jimerson DC. Testmeal response following m-Chlorophenylpiperazine and L-Tryptophan in bulimics and controls. Neuropsychopharmacology. 1994;11:63-71.

76. Mann J. Role of serotonergic system in the pathogenesis of major depression and suicidal behavior. Neuropsychopharmacology. 1999;21:99S-105S.

77. Okamoto Y, Okamoto Y, Kagaya A, et al. The relationship of the platelet 5-HT-induced calcium response to clinical symptoms in eating disorders. Psychopharmacology1999;142:289-94.

78. Collier DA, Arranz MJ, Li T, et al. Association between 5-HT$_{2A}$ gene promotor polymorphism and anorexia nervosa. Lancet. 1997;350:412.

79. Enoch M, Kaye WH, Rotondo A, et al. 5-HT$_{2A}$ promotor polymorphism–1438G/A, anorexia nervosa, and obsessive-compulsive disorder. Lancet. 1998;351:1785-6.

80. Sorbi S, Nacimas B, Tedde A, et al. 5-HT$_{2A}$ promotor polymorphism in anorexia nervosa. Lancet. 1998;351:1785.

81. Nacimas B, Ricca V, Tedde A, et al. 5-HT$_{2A}$ receptor gene polymorphisms in anorexia nervosa and bulimia nervosa. Neuroscience Letters. 1999;277:134-36.

82. Ricca V, Nacimas B, Cellini E, et al. 5HT$_{2A}$ receptor gene polymorphism and eating disorders. Neuroscience Letters. 2002;323:105-08.

83. Hinney A, Ziegler A, Nothen MM, et al. 5-HT$_{2A}$ receptor gene polymorphisms, anorexia nervosa, and obesity. Lancet. 1997; 350:1324-25.

84. Campbell DA, Sundaramurthy D, Markham AF, Pieri LF. Lack of association between 5-HT2A gene promotor polymorphism and susceptibility of anorexia nervosa. Lancet. 1998;352:499.

85. Karwautz A, Rabe-Hesketh S, Hu X, et al. Individual-specific risk factors for anorexia nervosa: A pilot study using a discordant sister-pair design. Psychol Med. 2001; 31:317-29.

86. Kipman A, Bruins-Slot L, Boni C, et al. 5-HT$_{2A}$ gene promoter polymorphism as a modifying rather than a vulnerability factor in anorexia nervosa. European Psychiatry. 2002;17:227-29.

87. Ziegler A, Hebebrand J, Gorg T, et al. Further lack of association between the 5-HT$_{2A}$ gene promotor polymorphism and susceptibility to eating disorders and a meta-analysis pertaining to anorexia nervosa. Molecular Psychiatry. 1999; 4:410-17.

88. Collier DA, Sham PC, Arranz MJ, Hu X, Treasure J. Understanding the genetic predisposition to anorexia nervosa. European Eating Disorders Review. 1999;7: 96-102.

89. Pieri LF, Campbell DA. Understanding the genetic predisposition to anorexia nervosa. European Eating Disorders Review. 1999;7:84-95.

90. Nishiguchi N, Matsushita S, Suzuki K, et al. Association between 5HT$_{2A}$ receptor gene promoter region polymorphism, and eating disorders in Japanese patients. Biol Psychiatry. 2001;50:123-28.

91. Eastwood H, Brown KMO, Markovic D, Pieri LF. Variation in the ESR1 and ESR2 genes and genetic susceptibility to anorexia nervosa. Molecular Psychiatry. 2002;7:86-89.

92. Rosenkranz K, Hinney A, Ziegler A, et al. Systematic mutation screening of the estrogen receptor beta gene in probands of different weight extremes: Identification of several genetic variants. J Clin Endocrinol Metab. 1998;83:4524-27.

93. Klump KL, McGue M, Iacono WG. Age differences in genetic and environmental influences on eating attitudes and behaviors in preadolescent and adolescent female twins. J Abnorm Psychol. 2000;109:239-51.

94. Klump KL, McGue M, Iacono WG. Differential heritability of eating pathology in pre-pubertal versus pubertal twins. Int J Eat Disord. 2003; 33(3):287-92.

95. Gorwood P, Ades J, Bellodi L, et al. The 5-HT$_{2a}$–1438G/A polymorphism is anorexia nervosa: A combined analysis of 316 trios from six European centres. Molecular Psychiatry. 2002;7:90-94.

96. Frisch A, Laufer N, Danziger Y, et al. Association of anorexia nervosa with the high activity allele of the COMT gene: A family-based study in Israeli patients. Molecular Psychiatry. 2001;6:243-45.

97. Koronyo-Hamaoui M, Danziger Y, Frisch A, et al. Association between anorexia nervosa and the hSKCa3 gene: A family-based case control study. Molecular Psychiatry. 2002;7:82-85.

98. Grice ED, Halmi KA, Fichter MM, et al. Evidence for susceptibility gene for anorexia nervosa on chromosome 1. Am J Hum Genet. 2002;70:787-92.

99. Bulik CM, Devlin B, Bacanu S-A, et al. Significant linkage on chromosome 10p in families with bulimia nervosa. Am J Hum Genet. 2003; 72(1):200-7.

100. Risch N, Merikangas KR. Linkage studies of psychiatric disorders. Eur Arch Psychiatry Clin Neurosci. 1993; 243:143-49.

101. Risch N, Merikangas K. The future of genetic studies of complex human diseases. Science. 1996; 73:1516-17.

102. Merikangas KR, Chakravarti A, Moldin SO, et al. Future of genetics of mood disorders research. Biol Psychiatry. 2002;52:457-77.

103. Sawa A, Snyder SH. Schizophrenia: Diverse approaches to a complex disease. Science. 2002;296:692-95.

104. Weatherall DJ. Single gene disorders or complex traits: Lessons from the thalessemias and other monogenic diseases. British Medical Journal. 2000;321: 1117-20.

105. Austin SB. Prevention research in eating disorders: Theory and new directions. Psychol Med. 2000;30:1249-62.

106. Keel PK, Mitchell JE. Outcome in bulimia nervosa. Am J Psychiatry. 1997; 154:313-21.

107. Steinhausen H. The outcome of anorexia nervosa in the 20th century. Am J Psychiatry. 2002;159:1284-93.

Body Mass Index and Alcohol Use

Katie D. Kleiner, BA
Mark S. Gold, MD
Kimberly Frost-Pineda, MPH
Barbra Lenz-Brunsman, MD
Michael G. Perri, PhD
William S. Jacobs, MD

SUMMARY. *Background.* Obesity, inactivity, and being overweight are leading causes of morbidity and mortality in the United States. The relationship between eating, overeating, and addiction have been discussed, debated, and more recently investigated. We have hypothesized that drugs of abuse compete with food for brain reward sites. Overeating and obesity may act as protective factors reducing drug reward and addiction.

Katie D. Kleiner is affiliated with the College of Medicine, University of Florida.

Mark S. Gold is affiliated with the University of Florida Departments of Psychiatry, Neuroscience, Community Health & Family Medicine, McKnight Brain Institute.

Kimberly Frost-Pineda is affiliated with the Department of Psychiatry, College of Medicine, University of Florida.

Barbra Lenz-Brunsman and Michael G. Perri are both affiliated with the Department of Clinical and Health Psychology, College of Health Professions, University of Florida.

William S. Jacob is affiliated with the Department of Psychiatry, College of Medicine, University of Florida.

Address all correspondence to: Mark S. Gold, MD, McKnight Brain Institute, P.O. Box 100183, Gainesville, FL 32610 (E-mail: msgold@psych.med.ufl.edu).

[Haworth co-indexing entry note]: "Body Mass Index and Alcohol Use." Kleiner, Katie D. et al. Co-published simultaneously in *Journal of Addictive Diseases* (The Haworth Medical Press, an imprint of The Haworth Press, Inc.) Vol. 23, No. 3, 2004, pp. 105-118; and: *Eating Disorders, Overeating, and Pathological Attachment to Food: Independent or Addictive Disorders?* (ed: Mark S. Gold) The Haworth Medical Press, an imprint of The Haworth Press, Inc., 2004, pp. 105-118. Single or multiple copies of this article are available for a fee from The Haworth Document Delivery Service [1-800-HAWORTH, 9:00 a.m. - 5:00 p.m. (EST). E-mail address: docdelivery@haworthpress.com].

http://www.haworthpress.com/web/JAD
© 2004 by The Haworth Press, Inc. All rights reserved.
Digital Object Identifer: 10.1300/J069v23n03_08

Methods. In the first part of this study, 374 charts of all active weight management patients in a 12-month period were examined. Demographic information, laboratory testing, psychiatric diagnostic interview, alcohol and drug history were reviewed. A detailed alcohol use, abuse, dependence history was present in 298 charts as part of the pre-bariatric evaluation. The relationship between BMI and alcohol use among female patients (n = 298) was then analyzed.

Results. We found a significant (p < .05) inverse relationship between BMI and alcohol consumption. The more obese the patient was, the less alcohol they consumed. The percentage of women who consumed alcohol in the past year decreased as BMI level increased. These results confirmed our surgeons' perception that it is rare to find a morbidly obese patient excluded for bariatric surgery because of excessive alcohol consumption.

Conclusions. Obese patients have lower rates of alcohol use than found in the general population of women. As BMI increases, lower rates of alcohol consumption are found. Overeating may compete with alcohol for brain reward sites, making alcohol ingestion less reinforcing. *[Article copies available for a fee from The Haworth Document Delivery Service: 1-800-HAWORTH. E-mail address: <docdelivery@haworthpress.com> Website: <http://www.HaworthPress.com> © 2004 by The Haworth Press, Inc. All rights reserved.]*

KEYWORDS. Alcohol, BMI, obesity, eating, addiction

INTRODUCTION

Obesity is a multi-factorial disease that is escalating in epidemic proportions nationally and internationally.[1] Recently, obesity has been identified as the most chronic health problem in the Western world.[2] According to the CDC, in 2000 nearly 39 million adults in the U.S. met the criteria for a diagnosis of obesity, defined as having a Body Mass Index score of 30 or more[3] (Table 1). From 1960 to1999, there was a significant increase in the number of overweight and obese adult Americans, increasing from 44% to 61%.[4,5] Moreover, the prevalence of obesity during this time more than doubled from 13% to 27%.[4,5]

These escalating rates have made obesity and being overweight leading causes of morbidity and mortality in the United States, second only to tobacco in the number of attributable deaths each year. The medical complications associated with obesity are significant and vast, including, but not limited to sleep apnea, hypertension, osteoarthritis, diabetes

TABLE 1. Body mass index table.

Body Mass Index Table

Height (inches)	Normal						Overweight					Obese										Extreme Obesity															
BMI	19	20	21	22	23	24	25	26	27	28	29	30	31	32	33	34	35	36	37	38	39	40	41	42	43	44	45	46	47	48	49	50	51	52	53	54
												Body Weight (pounds)																								
58	91	96	100	105	110	115	119	124	129	134	138	143	148	153	158	162	167	172	177	181	186	191	196	201	205	210	215	220	224	229	234	239	244	248	253	258
59	94	99	104	109	114	119	124	128	133	138	143	148	153	158	163	168	173	178	183	188	193	198	203	208	212	217	222	227	232	237	242	247	252	257	262	267
60	97	102	107	112	118	123	128	133	138	143	148	153	158	163	168	174	179	184	189	194	199	204	209	215	220	225	230	235	240	245	250	255	261	266	271	276
61	100	106	111	116	122	127	132	137	143	148	153	158	164	169	174	180	185	190	195	201	206	211	217	222	227	232	238	243	248	254	259	264	269	275	280	285
62	104	109	115	120	126	131	136	142	147	153	158	164	169	175	180	186	191	196	202	207	213	218	224	229	235	240	246	251	256	262	267	273	278	284	289	295
63	107	113	118	124	130	135	141	146	152	158	163	169	175	180	186	191	197	203	208	214	220	225	231	237	242	248	254	259	265	270	278	282	287	293	299	304
64	110	116	122	128	134	140	145	151	157	163	169	174	180	186	192	197	204	209	215	221	227	232	238	244	250	256	262	267	273	279	285	291	296	302	308	314
65	114	120	126	132	138	144	150	156	162	168	174	180	186	192	198	204	210	216	222	228	234	240	246	252	258	264	270	276	282	288	294	300	306	312	318	324
66	118	124	130	136	142	148	155	161	167	173	179	186	192	198	204	210	216	223	229	235	241	247	253	260	266	272	278	284	291	297	303	309	315	322	328	334
67	121	127	134	140	146	153	159	166	172	178	185	191	198	204	211	217	223	230	236	242	249	255	261	268	274	280	287	293	299	306	312	319	325	331	338	344
68	125	131	138	144	151	158	164	171	177	184	190	197	203	210	216	223	230	236	243	249	256	262	269	276	282	289	295	302	308	315	322	328	335	341	348	354
69	128	135	142	149	155	162	169	176	182	189	196	203	209	216	223	230	236	243	250	257	263	270	277	284	291	297	304	311	318	324	331	338	345	351	358	365
70	132	139	146	153	160	167	174	181	188	195	202	209	216	222	229	236	243	250	257	264	271	278	285	292	299	306	313	320	327	334	341	348	355	362	369	376
71	136	143	150	157	165	172	179	186	193	200	208	215	222	229	236	243	250	257	265	272	279	286	293	301	308	315	322	329	338	343	351	358	365	372	379	386
72	140	147	154	162	169	177	184	191	199	206	213	221	228	235	242	250	258	265	272	279	287	294	302	309	316	324	331	338	346	353	361	368	375	383	390	397
73	144	151	159	166	174	182	189	197	204	212	219	227	235	242	250	257	265	272	280	288	295	302	310	318	325	333	340	348	355	363	371	378	386	393	401	408
74	148	155	163	171	179	186	194	202	210	218	225	233	241	249	256	264	272	280	287	295	303	311	319	326	334	342	350	358	365	373	381	389	396	404	412	420
75	152	160	168	176	184	192	200	208	216	224	232	240	248	256	264	272	279	287	295	303	311	319	327	335	343	351	359	367	375	383	391	399	407	415	423	431
76	156	164	172	180	189	197	205	213	221	230	238	246	254	263	271	279	287	295	304	312	320	328	336	344	353	361	369	377	385	394	402	410	418	428	435	443

Source: Adapted from *Clinical Guidelines on the Identification, Evaluation, and Treatment of Overweight and Obesity in Adults: The Evidence Report.*

mellitus, gall bladder disease, heart disease, and other degenerative conditions including certain types of cancer.[6-19] Not surprisingly, the healthcare costs directly associated with obesity and these complications have also significantly increased and are presently estimated to be $70 billion or 9.4% of all health care costs.[20]

In order to comprehend this "so-called" epidemic, the relationship between eating, overeating, and addiction has been explored. Interestingly, some striking similarities have been discovered.[21] These findings suggest that eating for pleasure is distinct from eating when hungry and that in this way, food has the potential to act as a controlling substance. Consequently, we hypothesize that drugs of abuse can compete with food for brain reward sites, both ultimately providing the experience of pleasure. We have also noted that as a result of this relationship, overeating and obesity may act as protective factors reducing drug reward and addictions.

METHODS

In the first part of this study, charts of all weight management patients in a 12-month period were examined. Demographic data, BMI and substance use history were collected from 374 charts. We found severely obese patients with a Body Mass Index (BMI) of 55 or more were significantly less likely than those with a BMI of 45 or less to consume alcohol in the past year.[22] We then analyzed the relationship between BMI and alcohol use among female patients (n = 298) referred for weight management.

RESULTS

Mean age was 40.6 ± 11.64 years (range, 16 to 79). Mean BMI was 46.1 ± 11.8 kg/m² (range, 27 to 107) and mean initial weight was 276.4 ± 70 pounds (range 154 to 611). Analysis was done to compare four groups, those with BMI less than or equal to 29, those with a BMI from 30 through 39, from 40 through 49, and those with a BMI of 50 or more. We found an inverse relationship between BMI and alcohol consumption, such that the percentage of women who consumed alcohol in the past year decreased as BMI level increased. While 62.5% of the sample with BMI ≤ 29 (n = 8) used alcohol in the past year, only 47.6% of those with BMI 30-39 (n = 84), 41.8% of those with BMI 40-49 (n = 110), and only 35.4% (n = 96) of those with BMI ≥ 50 used alcohol in the past year. Pearson's correlation was −.115, p-value < .05. We concluded that alcohol use was significantly decreased for severely obese patients compared with previously collected telephone survey data within Florida and also national prevalence data (Figure 1).

DISCUSSION

Addiction

Addiction is a chronic disease that involves both biological and environmental variables.[23] Specifically it is characterized by compulsive self-administration without apparent regard to the consequences of consuming the addictive substance. The process of addiction is mediated

FIGURE 1. Past year alcohol use among obese women.

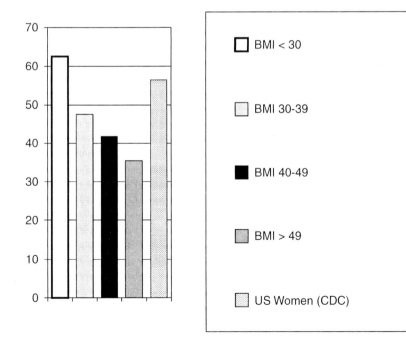

through brain mechanisms underlying reward or reinforcement. Reinforcement itself can be accomplished through both positive and negative mechanisms.

Addiction and the Human Brain

Recently, attempts to understand addiction and the way in which the biological and environmental factors interact have relied heavily on imaging studies such as positron emission tomography (PET) and functional magnetic resonance imaging (fMRI). Specifically these studies involve examining the neurochemical and functional changes in the brains of drug-addicted subjects.[24] The most impressive findings have shown that the reinforcing effects of frequently abused drugs are associated with large and rapid increases in dopamine.[24] Moreover, during drug withdrawal, the brain of an addict has significant deficits in dopamine function associated with deficits in the prefrontal regions. Since dopamine is additionally involved in the reinforcing effects of natural reinforcers, it has been suggested that this fluctuation in brain dopamine function subsequently decreases the sensitivity of natural reinforcers. Additionally, disruption in the frontal cortical functions may transpire which ultimately may result in disturbance in inhibitory control.

The functional imaging studies have proven that it is both drug craving and drug intoxication that cause direct dopaminergic activation of the brain circuitry involved in the reward (nucleus accumbens) pathway. The motivation (orbitofrontal cortex), memory (amygdala and hippocampus), and cognitive control (prefrontal cortex and cingulated gyrus) pathways also reveal some activation.[24] Thus, the consequence of chronic drug use is modification of multiple brain circuits in addition to loss of inhibitory control. This is believed to be the underlying mechanism which makes drugs of abuse addicting substances.[25,26]

Animal studies indicate that neurobiological mechanisms, which are involved in reinforcement, do in fact promote certain behaviors. Dopamine D2 receptor levels mediate reinforcing responses to drugs of abuse such that there is a decrease in the reinforcing effects of alcohol and morphine in mice that lack dopamine D2 receptors.[27,28] Moreover, the animal studies have shown a decrease in the reinforcing effects of cocaine in animals whose dopamine D2 receptors are blocked.

The human studies, however, are not as transparent. For example, whereas the mice show a reduction in self-administration of alcohol when given a dopamine agonist, humans show no effect when given long-acting bromocriptine, a D(2) agonist. This suggests the complexity of dependence-related behaviors in humans.[29]

Neurobiological Theories of Etiology of Obesity

Eating for Pleasure

Like many illicit drugs, anticipation and ingestion of food causes an increase in the extracellular level of dopamine in the nucleus accumbens, a major target of the mesolimbic dopaminergic system.[30-35] It is in this way that eating behaviors can mimic addiction behaviors. In effect, the brain does not seem to differentiate whether the reward is provoked by licit or illicit drugs or extreme environmental manipulations or fasting.

There is a significant amount of research suggesting that it is this reinforcing dopaminergic neurotransmission that may be involved in obesity. Specifically, there is a high prevalence of the Taq I A allele for the dopamine D2 receptors in obese subjects.[36] This Taq I A allele has itself been linked with lower levels of dopamine D2 receptors.[37] Thus individuals with the A1 allele may use food to elevate dopamine stimulation and subsequently, the reinforcement desired.[38] These findings suggest that this is the likely mechanism by which low dopamine brain activity may contribute to dysfunctional eating behaviors.

Additional research supporting this theory has been provided by positron emission tomography (PET) and [11c]raclopride, which both measure dopamine D2 receptor levels. Studies have shown that obese subjects have significantly lower amounts of striatal dopamine D2 receptor availability than control subjects.[39] Given that dopamine D2 receptors mediate reinforcing responses, these findings suggest that obesity reflects a "reward deficiency syndrome."[40] Since dopamine has a role in regulating food intake by modulating food reward via the meso-limbic circuitry and nucleus accumbens, it is suspected that dopamine D2 receptors regulate compulsiveness in pathological eaters. Additional studies are needed to determine if low dopamine D2 levels are associated with obesity due to the fact that they contribute to a higher vulnerability for addictive behaviors or if there is another neurobiological mechanism at play.

Animal studies have further demonstrated the similarities and relationship between illicit drugs and food. Carroll[41] and Specker and colleagues[42] showed that rats self administer drugs too a much greater extent when they are food deprived.[41,42] Furthermore, studies using rhesus monkeys have revealed that non-drug alternative reinforcers, such as saccharin, reduce drug self-administration.[43] These findings have been replicated with phencyclidine (PCP)[41,44-46] ethanol,[47] and smoked cocaine base.[48] Human studies have noted that other non-drug reinforcers, such as material items and money, work in a similar fashion and, when available, result in a reduction in drug self-administration.[49-52]

PET and 2-deoxy-2-[^{18}F]fluro-D-glucose have also been used in human subjects to assess whether or not obese subjects have an enhanced sensitivity in the brain region associated with sensory processing of food.[53] It was found that, in fact, obese subjects did have significantly greater glucose metabolism in the postcentral gyrus of the left and right parietal cortex.[53] This is where the somatosensory maps of the mouth, lips, and tongue are located and it is also the area in which taste perception occurs. The increased activity in these regions may explain how food is more rewarding and thus, more salient to obese individuals.

Several laboratory animal and human studies have examined factors that influence the choice between eating or engaging in alternative behaviors.[54-58] These studies have shown that, like other reinforcers, eating is subject to the same factors such as the amount of work required to obtain the reinforcer, the quantity and timing of consumption of the reinforcer, and the alternative activities available other than eating.[54-58]

The relative reinforcing value of eating food as opposed to engaging in alternative activities can be determined by providing subjects the opportunity to work for access to the alternatives. The relative reinforcing value is determined based on the amount of work done to obtain one vs. another alternative. Overwhelmingly, the studies show that whichever alternative the subject works harder for, the more rewarding that alternative is. Johnson found that obese subjects consumed more calories and worked harder to obtain food than non-obese subjects when food cues were visible during a food-directed reinforcement task.[59] Similar findings include that overweight adults reporting a higher reinforcement value for eating on reinforcement surveys compared to adults who were not overweight.[59,60]

Eating Due to Hunger

Neuropeptide Y (NPY), agouti related peptide (AgrP) and γ-aminobutyric acid (GABA) are other neuromodulators that promote feeding behavior. These substances, however, seem to be related to the appetitive drive due to hunger as opposed to pleasure. Nevertheless, disturbances in these substances, may also play a role in the pathological eating behaviors that lead to obesity.

NPY stimulates food intake by activation of NPY Y1 and Y5 receptors in the medial paraventricular nucleus.[61] Studies show that hyperphagia, increased rates of body weight gain, and ultimately morbid obesity result when there is continuous stimulation of NPY receptors.[61,62] Moreover both fasting and dieting readily increased NPY synthesis in the arcuate nucleus (ARC) and release in the paraventricular nucleus (PVN) to sustain the appetitive drive needed for energy replenishment.[62,63] Interestingly, reduction in NPY availability at target sites in the PVN and possibly in the ARC enhanced NPY Y1 receptor sensitivity resulting in hyperphagia among these rats and overt obesity.[62,64] Thus, it appears that an imbalance in NPY signaling locally in the ARC and PVN results in unregulated phagia involving distinctive molecular sequalae.[65]

GABA has been shown to stimulate feeding via GABA^A receptor activation or locally in the ARC itself, which reduces anorexigenic melanocortin signaling to the PVN, resulting in enhanced feeding.[66]

AgrP, an endogenous antagonist at melanocortin 4 (MC4) receptors, stimulates feeding by a distinct mode of signal relay in the PVN. The MC4 receptors mediate the tonic restraint on feeding.[61,67,68]

Additionally, the neuromodulators α-MSH and cocaine-and-amphetamine regulating transcript (CART) are involved in promoting satiety and inhibiting feeding, and therefore, disturbances of these also have the potential to be involved in obesity. These peptides are released in the PVN where they act to inhibit feeding.[61,66,69] The inhibitatory effects of α-MSH are mediated by MC4 receptors, the same receptors which normally mediate the tonic restraint on feeding. In fact, studies have shown that mice with a null mutation for MC4 receptors develop hyperphagia and obesity.[61,66,70]

It is important to note that Pirola and Lieber reported on the hypermetabolic effect of alcohol more than thirty years ago, however this applies only to higher consumption rates.[71,72] In their study, Pirola and Lieber found that when a group of alcoholics had fifty percent of carbohydrate calories replaced with ethanol, a small but significant decrease in body weight was noted.[71] They also compared adding 2000 kcal/day of ethanol or chocolate to the diet. The additional calories from chocolate resulted in significant weight gain (approximately six pounds in two week), however mean change in weight with the additional calories from ethanol, even after 30 days, was less than half a pound.[71] In a later paper, they describe the possible role of hepatic microsomal enzymes in the energy wastage found in alcoholism.[72]

CONCLUSIONS

Obese female patients (BMI $\geq$ 30) have lower rates of alcohol use than found in the general population of women (56.4% recently reported by the CDC).[73] As BMI increases, lower rates of alcohol consumption are found. Conversely, BMI increases during supervised abstinence.[74] Overeating may compete with alcohol for brain reward sites and result in reduced alcohol intake and dependence rates. Drugs of abuse may hijack existing reward pathways as suggested by Volkow and others,[24] but of these pathways, the food pathways are primary.

REFERENCES

1. Mokdad AH, Serdula MK, Dietz WH, Bowman BA, Marks JS, Koplan JP. The spread of obesity epidemic in the United States, 1991-1998. *JAMA*. 1999; 282:1519-1522.

2. O'Brien PE, Dixon JB. Laparoscopic adjustable gastric banding in the treatment of morbid obesity. *Arch Surg*. 2003;138(4):376-382.

3. Centers for Disease Control. Obesity Trends. Available online at http://www.cdc.gov/nccdphp/dnpa/obesity/trend/index.htm. Accessed July 8, 2003.

4. Frank A. Futility and avoidance. Medical professionals in the treatment of obesity. *JAMA* 1993;269:2132-2133.

5. McTigue KM, Garrett JM, Popkin BM. The natural history of the development of obesity in a cohort of young U.S. adults between 1981 and 1998. *Annals of Internal Medicine* 2002;136:857-864.

6. Allison DB, Fontaine KR, Manson JE, Stevens J, VanItallie TB. Annual deaths attributable to obesity in the United States. *JAMA*. 1999;282:1530-1538.

7. Must A, Spadano J, Coakley EH, Field AE, Colditz G, Dietz WH. The disease burden associated with overweight and obesity. *JAMA*. 1999;282:1523-1529.

8. Allison DB, Zannolli R, Narayan KM. The direct health care costs of obesity in the United States. *Am J Public Health*. 1999;89:1194-1199.

9. Bray GA. Complications of obesity. *Ann Intern Med*. 1985;103:1052-1062.

10. Bray GA. Health hazards of obesity. *Endocrinol Metab Clin North Am*. 1996; 25:907-919.

11. Calle EE, Rodriguez C, Walker-Thurmond K, Thun MJ. Overweight, obesity, and mortality from cancer in a prospectively studied cohort of U.S. adults. *NEJM*. 2003;348:1625-1638.

12. Calle EE, Thun MJ, Petrelli JM, Rodriguez C, Heath CW Jr. Body-mass index and mortality in a prospective cohort of US adults. *NEJM*. 1999;341:1097-1105.

13. Manson JE, Willett WC, Stampfer MJ, et al. Body weight and mortality among women [see "Comment" section]. *NEJM.* 1995;333:677-685.

14. Pi-Sunyer FX. Medical hazards of obesity. *Ann Intern Med.* 1993;119:655-660.

15. Quesenberry CP Jr, Caan B, Jacobson A. Obesity, health services use, and health care costs among members of a health maintenance organization. *Arch Intern Med.* 1998;158:466-472.

16. Stevens J, Cai J, Pamuk ER, Williamson DF, Thun MJ, Wood JL. The effect of age on the association between body-mass index and mortality [see "Comment" section]. *NEJM.* 1998;338:1-7.

17. Thompson D, Edelsberg J, Colditz GA, Bird AP, Oster G. Lifetime health and economic consequences of obesity. *Arch Intern Med.* 1999;159:2177-2183.

18. National Institute of Health News Release. First Federal Obesity Clinical Guidelines Released. 1998. Available online at http://www.nhlbi.nih.gov/error_messages/nhlbi.htm. Accessed on July 22, 2003.

19. Stunkard AJ, Wadden TA, eds. Obesity Theory and Therapy. New York: Raven Press; 1993:179-195.

20. Livingston EH, Fink AS. Quality of life: Cost and future of bariatric surgery. *Arch Surg.* 2003;138(4):383-388. Review.

21. Gold MS, Frost-Pineda K, Jacobs, WS. Overeating, binge eating, and eating disorders as addictions. *Psych Annals.* 2003;33(2):117-122.

22. Jacobs WS, Perri M, Gold MS, Frost-Pineda K, Lenz-Brunsman, B. Body mass index and alcohol use. *Biol Psych.* 2003;53:16.

23. Leshner AI. Addiction is a brain disease, and it matters. *Science.* 1997;278:45-47.

24. Volkow ND, Fowler JS, Wang G. The addicted human brain: insights from imaging studies. *Journal of Clinical Investigation.* 2003;111:1444-1451.

25. Chiara GD. Nucleus accumbens shell and core dopamine: Differential role in behavior and addiction. *Behavioural Brain Research.* 2002;137:75-114.

26. Wise RA. Neuroleptics and operant behavior: The anhedonia hypothesis. *Behav Brain Sci.* 1982;5:39-87.

27. Phillips, RG, Hill, AJ. Fat, plain, but not friendless: Self-esteem and peer acceptance of obese pre-adolescent girls. *Int J Obes Relat Metab Disord.* 1998;22: 287-293.

28. Maldonado R, Saiardi A, Valverde O, Samad TA, Roques BP, Borrelli E. Absence of opiate rewarding effects in mice lacking dopamine D2 receptors. *Nature* 1997; 388:586-589.

29. Naranjo CA, Chu AY, Tremblay LK. Neurodevelopmental liabilities in alcohol dependence: Central serotonin and dopamine dysfunction. *Neurotox Res.* 2002;4(4): 343-361.

30. Hernandez L, Hoebel B. Feeding and hypothalamic stimulation increase dopamine turnover in the accumbens. *Physio Behav.* 1988;44:599-606.

31. Hernandez L, Hoebel BG. Feeding can enhance dopamine turnover in the prefrontal cortex. *Brain Res Bull.* 1990;25:975-979.

32. Mogenson GJ. Studies of the nucleus accumbens and its mesolimbic dopaminergic affects in relation to ingestive behaviors and reward. In: Hoebel GB, Novin D, eds. The Neural Basis of Feeding and Reward. Brunswick, ME. Haer Institute; 1982: 275-506.

33. Radhakishun FS, van Ree JM, Westerink BH. Scheduled eating increases dopamine release in the nucleus accumbens of food-deprived rats as assessed with on-line dialysis. *Neuroscience Letters* 1988;85:351-356.

34. Yoshida M Yokoo H, Mizoguchi K, et al. Eating and drinking cause increased dopamine release in the nucleus accumbens and ventral tegmental area in the rat: measurement by in vivo microdialysis. *Neurosci Lett.* 1992;139:73-76.

35. Young AM, Joseph MN, Gray JA. Increased dopamine release in vivo in nucleus accumbens an caudate nucleus of the rat during drinking: A microdialysis study. *Neuroscience* 1992;48:871-876.

36. Noble EP, Noble RE, Ritchie T, et al. D2 dopamine receptor gene and obesity. *Int J Eat Disord.* 1994;15:205-217.

37. Noble EP, Blum K, Ritchie T, et al. Allelic association of the D2 dopamine receptor gene with receptor-binding characteristics in alcoholism. *Arch Gen Psychiatry* 1991;48:648-654.

38. Noble EP, Fitch RJ, Ritchie T, et al. The D2 dopamine receptor gene: Obesity, smoking and mood. In: St. Jeor ST, Koop CE, eds. Obesity Assessment: Tools, Methods, Interpretations. New York, NY: Chapman and Hall; 1997:522-533.

39. Wang GJ, Volkow ND, Logan J, et al. Brain dopamine and obesity. *Lancet* 2001;357:354-357.

40. Blum K, Cull JG, Braverman ER, Comings DE. Reward deficiency syndrome. *American Scientist* 1996;84:132-145.

41. Carroll ME. Concurrent phencyclidine and saccharin access: presentation of an alternative reinforcer reduces drug intake. *J Exp Anal Behav.* 1985;43:131-144.

42. Specker SM, Lac ST, Carroll ME. Food deprivation history and cocaine self-administration: An animal model of binge eating. *Pharmacol Biochem Behav.* 1994;48(4): 1025-1029.

43. Campbell UC, Carroll ME. Reduction of drug self-administration by an alternative non-drug reinforcer in rhesus monkeys: Magnitude and temporal effects. *Psychopharmacology (Berl).* 2000;147: 418-425.

44. Carroll ME, Carmona GG, May SA. Modifying drug-reinforced behavior by altering the economic conditions of the drug and a nondrug reinforcer. *J Exp Anal Behav.* 1991;56:361-376.

45. Carroll ME, Rodefer JS. Income alters choice between drug and an alternative nondrug reinforcer in monkeys. *Exp Clin Psychopharm* 1993;1:10-120.

46. Rodefer JS, Carroll ME. A comparison of progressive ratio schedules versus behavioral economic measures: Effect of an alternative reinforcer on the reinforcing efficacy of phencyclidine. *Psychopharmacology* 1997;132:95-103.

47. Carroll ME, Rodefer JS, Rawleigh JM. Concurrent self-administration of ethanol and an alternative nondrug reinforcer in monkeys: Effects of income (session length) on demand for drug. *Psychopharmacology* 1995;120:1-9.

48. Comer SD, Hunt VR, Carroll ME. Effects of concurrent saccharin availability and buprenorphine pretreatment on demand for smoked cocaine base in rhesus monkeys. *Psychopharmacology* 1994;115:15-23.

49. Higgins ST, Budney AJ, Bickel WK, Hughes JR, Foerg BA, Badger G. Achieving cocaine abstinence with a behavioral approach. *Am J Psychiatry* 1993;150:763-769.

50. Zacny JP, Divane WT, de Wit H. Assessment of magnitude and availability of a non-drug reinforcer on preference for a drug reinforcer. *Hum Psychopharmacol.* 1992; 7:281-286.

51. Foltin RW, Fischman MW. Cocaine self-administration research: Treatment implications. *NIDA Res Monogr.* 1994;145:139-162.

52. Hatsukami DK, Thompson TN, Pentel PR, Flygare BK, Carroll ME. Self-administration of smoked cocaine. *Exp Clin Psychopharm.* 1994;2:115-125.

53. Wang GJ, Volkow ND, Fowler JS, et al. Enhanced resting activity of the somatosensory cortex in obese subjects. *Neuroreport.* 2002;13:1151-1155.

54. Foltin RW. An economic analysis of "demand" for food in baboons. *Journal of the Experimental Analysis of Behavior.* 1991;56:445-454.

55. Foltin RW Economic analysis of the eVects of caloric alternatives and reinforcer magnitude on "demand" for food in baboons. *Appetite.* 1992;19:255-271.

56. Foltin RW, Fischman MW. The effects of varying procurement costs on food intake in baboons. *Physiology and Behavior.* 1988;43:493-499.

57. Lappalainen R, Epstein LH. A behavioral economics analysis of food choice in humans. *Appetite.* 1990;14:81-93.

58. Smith JA, Epstein LH. Behavioral economic analysis of food choice in obese children. *Appetite* 1991;17:91-95.

59. Johnson WG. Effect of cue prominence and subject weight on human food-directed performance. *Journal of Personality and Social Psychology* 1974;29:843-848.

60. Jacobs SB, Wagner MK. Obese and nonobese individuals: Behavioral and personality characteristics. *Addictive Behaviors.* 1984;9:223-226.

61. Kalra SP, Dube MG, Pu S, Xu B, Horvath TL, Kalra PS. Interacting appetite-regulating pathways in the hypothalamic regulation of body weight. *Endocr Rev.* 1999;20:68-100.

62. Kalra SP, Kalra PS. Nutritional infertility: The role of the interconnected hypothalamic neuropeptide Y-galanin-opioid network. *Front Neuroendocrinol.* 1996;17: 371-401.

63. Kalra SP, Dube MG, Sahu A, Phelps, CP, Kalra PS. Neuropeptide Y secretion increases in the paraventricular nucleus in association with increased appetite for food. *Proc Natl Acad Sci USA* 1991;88:10931-10935.

64. Kalra PS, Dube MG, Xu B, Kalra SP. Increased receptor sensitivity to neuropeptide Y in the hypothalamus may underlie transient hyperphagia and body weight gain. *Regul Pept.* 1997;72:121-130.

65. Kalra SP, Kalra PS. Overlapping and interactive pathways regulating appetite and craving. *Journal of Addictive* 2004;23(3):5-21.

66. Cowley MA, Smart JL, Rubinstein M, Cerdan MG, Diano S, Horvath TL, Cone RD, Low MJ. Leptin activates anorexigenic POMC neurons through a neural network in the arcuate nucleus. *Nature* 2001;411:480-484.

67. Ollmann MM, Wilson BD, Yang YK, Kerns JA, Chen Y, Gantz I, Barsh GS. Antagonism of central melanocortin receptors in vitro and in vivo by agouti-related protein. *Science* 1997;278:135-138.

68. Hahn TM, Breininger JF, Baskin DG, Schwartz MW. Coexpression of Agrp and NPY in fasting-activated hypothalamic neurons. *Nat Neurosci.* 1998;1:271-272.

69. Broberger C, Hokfelt T. Hypothalamic and vagal neuropeptide circuitries regulating food intake. *Physiol Behav.* 2001;74:669-682.

70. Saper CB, Chou TC, Elmquist JK. The need to feed: Homeostatic and hedonic control of eating. *Neuron* 2002;36:199-211.

71. Pirola RC, Lieber CS. The energy cost of the metabolism of drugs, including ethanol. *Pharmacology* 1972;7:185-196.

72. Pirola RC, Lieber CS. Hypothesis: Energy wastage in alcoholism and drug abuse: Possible role of hepatic microsomal enzymes. *Am J Clin Nutr.* 1976;29:90-93.

73. Schoenborn CA, Adams FA. Alcohol use among adults: United States, 1997-98. Advance Data From Vital and Health Statistics. CDC 2002.

74. Hodgkins CC, Cahill KS, Seraphine AE, Frost-Pineda K, Gold MS. Adolescent drug addiction treatment and weight gain. *J Addict Dis.* 2004;23(3):55-65.

Index

BOOK ORDER FORM!

Order a copy of this book with this form or online at:
http://www.haworthpress.com/store/product.asp?sku=5336

Eating Disorders, Overeating, and Pathological Attachment to Food
Independent or Addictive Disorders?

____ in softbound at $19.95 (ISBN: 0-7890-2600-7)
____ in hardbound at $34.95 (ISBN: 0-7890-2593-0)

COST OF BOOKS _____

POSTAGE & HANDLING _____
US: $4.00 for first book & $1.50
for each additional book
Outside US: $5.00 for first book
& $2.00 for each additional book.

SUBTOTAL _____

In Canada: add 7% GST. _____

STATE TAX _____
CA, IL, IN, MN, NY, OH & SD residents
please add appropriate local sales tax.

FINAL TOTAL _____
If paying in Canadian funds, convert
using the current exchange rate,
UNESCO coupons welcome.

❏ BILL ME LATER:
Bill-me option is good on US/Canada/
Mexico orders only; not good to jobbers,
wholesalers, or subscription agencies.

❏ Signature _____

❏ Payment Enclosed: $ _____

❏ PLEASE CHARGE TO MY CREDIT CARD:
❏ Visa ❏ MasterCard ❏ AmEx ❏ Discover
❏ Diner's Club ❏ Eurocard ❏ JCB

Account # _____

Exp Date _____

Signature _____
(Prices in US dollars and subject to change without notice.)

PLEASE PRINT ALL INFORMATION OR ATTACH YOUR BUSINESS CARD

Name

Address

City   State/Province   Zip/Postal Code

Country

Tel   Fax

E-Mail

May we use your e-mail address for confirmations and other types of information? ❏ Yes ❏ No We appreciate receiving
your e-mail address. Haworth would like to e-mail special discount offers to you, as a preferred customer.
We will never share, rent, or exchange your e-mail address. We regard such actions as an invasion of your privacy.

Order From Your **Local Bookstore** or Directly From
The Haworth Press, Inc. 10 Alice Street, Binghamton, New York 13904-1580 • USA
Call Our toll-free number (1-800-429-6784) / Outside US/Canada: (607) 722-5857
Fax: 1-800-895-0582 / Outside US/Canada: (607) 771-0012
E-mail your order to us: orders@haworthpress.com

For orders outside US and Canada, you may wish to order through your local
sales representative, distributor, or bookseller.
For information, see http://haworthpress.com/distributors

(Discounts are available for individual orders in US and Canada only, not booksellers/distributors.)

Please photocopy this form for your personal use.
www.HaworthPress.com

BOF04